THE 7-DAY
HAY DIET PLAN

CAROLYN HUMPHRIES

foulsham
LONDON • NEW YORK • TORONTO • SYDNEY

foulsham

The Publishing House, Bennetts Close,
Cippenham, Slough, Berks SL1 5AP, England

ISBN 0-572-02406-1

Cover photograph © The Image Bank

Text illustrations by Sophie Azimont

Printed in Great Britain by Cox & Wyman Ltd, Reading, Berks

CONTENTS

Introduction

Do you feel flabby, overweight or generally sluggish and uninspired? Your diet could be your problem. If you tend to pig out on junk food – or find yourself raiding the biscuit tin several times a day – you won't know what it's like to have a really healthy body. When you eat well – and wisely – you feel exhilarated, energetic, vibrant, happy. Your brain can function at its peak and your body too. That doesn't mean starving yourself, it means eating three meals a day plus snacks. But it's what you eat and when that matters.

Food combining is a complete lifestyle, not a cranky slimming diet. You call the tune, choosing what foods you eat and how much in a mix 'n' match fashion. After a while it will become second nature to know what to eat with what and what to avoid. It's not difficult. In the next few pages you'll discover the few simple guidelines you need to follow, then there is a whole wealth of simple but delicious recipes for every occasion.

If you need to lose weight, you'll find this the ideal 'diet'. You get to eat filling 'real' food, not just a lettuce leaf and a glass of tomato juice – and no need to calorie count. If you are underweight food combining will help, too. Because it makes your digestive system work properly, you will absorb more nutrients from your food and so become more healthy. Or if you just feel you are underfunctioning and in need of a 'lift', this book could change your life. Once you've experienced food combining for just 28 days, using the supplied menu guide or combining meals yourself – and the hints on weight loss or gain if you need to – you'll look and feel like a new person.

WHAT IS
FOOD COMBINING?

Food combining means only eating foods that harmonise together so the digestive system can work with optimum efficiency. It is a very simple system once you have mastered the technique.

The American Dr William Howard Hay discovered this way of eating to treat his own serious kidney condition. He originally called it food separation. But as it isn't possible to separate foods completely, the term food combining was adopted. All it means is that you don't mix starches and sugars (carbohydrates) with proteins and acid fruits at the same meal.

The Simple Rules

❦ Vegetables and salads should form the major part of the diet (three parts vegetables and salad to one part protein OR carbohydrate).

❦ Never mix foods from the protein group with foods from the carbohydrate group at the same meal.

❦ Proteins, carbohydrates and fats should be eaten in small quantities.

❦ Foods from the neutral group can be eaten with foods from the protein group or the carbohydrate group.

❦ Only wholegrain and unprocessed starches should be eaten (see carbohydrate foods page 14).

❦ Avoid processed foods such as white flour, sugars and margarine.

❦ Avoid smoked products and processed meats, such as sausages.

❦ Fruit should generally be eaten raw and ripe, combining acid fruits such as oranges with proteins and sweet fruits such as bananas with carbohydrates or eat them on their own as a snack between meals. Dried fruits and bananas may be eaten cooked occasionally.

❦ Drink plenty – at least 1 litre/1¾ pts/4¼ cups of fluid a day – including lots of mineral water (see Foods To Avoid page 18).

❦ Ideally have four hours between meals so don't eat the snacks between meals unless genuinely hungry!

❦ It's an excellent idea to start and end your day with a glass of hot or cold mineral water with a slice of lemon in it.

❦ Don't drink too much with your meals. You need to chew and salivate as much as possible and gulping down food with liquid inhibits this. At most, sip a glass of mineral water with any meal. If you want to have alcohol, choose wine or cider with a protein meal and beer with a carbohydrate one – and remember to keep it in moderation! For breakfast, finish your meal with a cup of herb tea. If you must have tea or coffee, make it decaffeinated and drink it with cream.

Weight Loss

This eating plan should make you lose excess body weight anyway. But if you want to lose a substantial amount, you can still enjoy three good meals every day and snacks in between, but here are a few useful tips.

❦ Stick to a piece of fruit from the protein group, such as an apple, orange or peach mid-morning and a banana or handful of raisins, from the carbohydrate group, mid-afternoon.

❦ Go very easy on fats. Have just a mere scraping of butter on bread. Don't go overboard with too many cream recipes either. For instance, if a serving suggestion is strawberries and cream, you're better off leaving out the cream and just enjoying the fruit. Keep oil to a minimum for cooking or for dressing salads. Grill (broil) rather than fry (sauté) foods whenever possible.

❦ Choose skimmed milk and very low fat yoghurt.

❦ Choose reduced fat hard cheeses and low-fat soft cheeses.

❦ Drink plenty of mineral water.

❦ Always fill up on more neutral vegetables or salad.

Weight Gain

If you are underweight, this eating plan should help you become better nourished. Try to eat all the snacks and desserts suggested in the menu plan – that is, a protein snack mid-morning and a carbohydrate snack mid-afternoon but make sure you eat masses of neutral vegetables and salad every day which is most important.

Which Foods Are Which?

The Food Combining Plan on page 12 will tell you exactly which foods belong to the protein group, which fall into the carbohydrate group and which are the neutral foods. It also gives you a list of foods which are best avoided altogether.

The neutral foods can be mixed in a meal with foods from the protein or carbohydrate group or on their own. The neutral foods harmonise with all foods and will not disrupt the digestive system at all. You may find some of the neutral listings a bit confusing, but I assure you they are based on years of experience. For example, soured milk products are neutral because, although they are full of protein, the protein has been changed in the souring and is therefore easier to digest.

All fats are neutral because they are digested in the duodenum, not the stomach, so they do not interfere with the digestion of other foods. But you should keep their intake to a minimum and avoid processed fats such as margarine. Use butter or naturally produced oils such as cold-pressed olive oil. A high fat intake is not recommended, so avoid frying or roasting in fat where possible – especially if you wish to lose weight. Full-fat cream cheese, such as Mascarpone, is also neutral, but other cheeses come in to the protein group.

Family Meals

If the rest of the family don't wish to join you on the diet, it's no problem. Simply supplement your meals for them. Add meat, fish, eggs or cheese to any of your carbohydrate-rich meals or add potatoes, rice, pasta or bread to any protein-rich one (but don't be tempted to have any yourself!). When they're feeling over-full and ready for a snooze, you'll be feeling fresh, fit and raring to go!

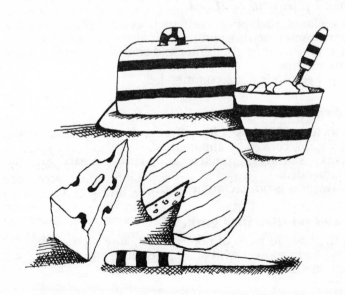

THE FOOD COMBINING PLAN

Within one meal, foods belonging to the protein group should not be mixed with those from the carbohydrate group. So at any meal you should have either:

Foods from the protein and neutral groups

OR

Foods from the carbohydrate and neutral groups

OR

Foods just from the neutral group.

Ideally have one protein-rich, one carbohydrate-rich and one completely neutral meal each day.

Protein Group

Cooked fish and seafood

This includes all types of fish such as cod, plaice, salmon, tuna, mackerel, herring and trout. It also includes all seafood such as prawns, mussels, lobster and crab in any form, cooked by any method.

Smoked fish is not recommended.

Cooked meat

This includes all types of lean meat such as beef, lamb or veal in any form, cooked by any method.

Pork, sausages, smoked and cured meats are not recommended.

Raw meat is not recommended.

Cooked poultry and game

This includes all types of poultry and game such as chicken, turkey, duck, goose, rabbit and pheasant in any form, cooked by any method.

Milk and milk products

This includes milk of all fat levels, yoghurt, fromage frais and quark.

Cream and crème fraîche are neutral foods.

Milk combines best with fruit and should not be served with meat.

Whole cooked eggs

Egg yolks on their own are a neutral food.

Raw egg white is not recommended.

Cheese

This includes all kinds of cheese from hard cheeses like Parmesan, Emmental, Stilton or Cheddar to soft cheeses like Brie, Camembert, Dolcelatte and Mozzarella. It also includes cottage, curd and low-, medium- and full-fat soft cheeses.

Full-fat cream cheese like Mascarpone has such a low protein content that it is classed as a neutral food so can be used to top jacket potatoes for example. Check the label: it should have around 5 per cent protein. If in any doubt about any cheese you are using, class it as a protein food.

Cooked or canned tomatoes

Raw, fresh tomatoes are in the neutral group.

Berry fruit

This includes blackberries, blueberries, gooseberries, loganberries, strawberries and raspberries.

Cranberries are not recommended.

Citrus fruit

This includes oranges, clementines, satsumas, grapefruit, limes, lemons, uglis and tangerines.

Hard fruit

This includes apples, crisp pears and pineapples.

Rhubarb (which is really a vegetable) is not recommended.

Exotic fruit

This includes guavas, kiwi fruit, lychees, mangoes, passion fruit and pomegranates.

Melon should be eaten alone as a fruit meal.

Bananas, very sweet papayas and pears, figs and dates are classed as carbohydrates.

Stone fruit

This includes apricots, cherries, sharp grapes, peaches and nectarines.

All fruit should generally be eaten raw, not cooked.

Plums are not recommended.

Dried cake fruits like raisins are classed as carbohydrates.

Fruit drinks

These include all drinks made with fruit such as fruit teas, fruit juices, white, red, rosé and sparkling wine and cider. They also include lemon and lime juice used for flavouring.

Vinegar is not recommended.

Soya products

This includes soy sauce, tofu, TVP (soya protein) and sandwich spreads made from soya.

TIP

◆ Do not use breadcrumbs for coating foods from the protein group. Use sesame (or other) seeds, or ground or chopped nuts instead.

Carbohydrate Group

Cereals

This includes wheat, rye, barley, oats, millet, maize, buckwheat and brown rice.

Refined white rice is not recommended.

Wholemeal cereal products

This includes bread, biscuits and cakes made from wholemeal flour, wholemeal pasta and wholemeal semolina.

Refined white flour and white flour products like white bread and pasta, cakes and sweet and savoury biscuits are not recommended.

TIP

◆ Cereal rissoles and potato cakes should be coated in wholemeal breadcrumbs or sesame seeds, not in beaten egg or milk first. If you must use something to make the coating 'stick' use a little cream or beaten egg yolk only.

Starchy powders

These include most thickening agents like cornflour (cornstarch), arrowroot, potato flour, custard powder and carob powder.

Cocoa (unsweetened chocolate) powder is not recommended.

Non-acid fruits

This includes bananas, fresh dates and figs, very sweet dessert grapes, pears (if very ripe) and papaya (if very soft and ripe).

TIP

◆ If in doubt that pears, grapes or papaya are ripe enough, don't include.

Dried fruit

Currants, sultanas (golden raisins), raisins, dates, figs, bananas, pears and prunes (not too often!).

Dried apricots, apples and pineapple are protein.

Starchy vegetables

These include Jerusalem artichokes, potatoes (best eaten with the skins on), pumpkin, marrow (squash), salsify, sweetcorn (corn), sweet potatoes and yams.

Beer

Sweeteners

Honey, pure maple syrup (not maple-flavoured syrup), natural fruit syrup.

Refined sugar and sugar products such as jam, marmalade, golden (light corn) syrup and glucose are not recommended.

Neutral Group

Foods from this group can be mixed with foods from the protein or carbohydrate groups or served on their own. Examples and exceptions are listed under each item.

Fats

Butter or naturally produced oils such as cold-pressed olive oil, sunflower, sesame or walnut oil.

Processed fats such as margarine and other 'bread spreads' are not recommended. Avoid white fats such as lard, too.

Soured milk products

Soured (dairy sour) cream, crème fraîche and buttermilk.

Cream

Single (light), whipping and double (heavy) cream.

Cream cheese

Full-fat cream varieties such as Mascarpone.

Vegetables

These include all green, yellow and red varieties such as asparagus, aubergines (eggplants), green beans, beetroot (red beet), broccoli, Brussels sprouts, cabbage and greens (all types), carrots, cauliflower, celery, celeriac (celery root), courgettes (zucchini), fennel, globe artichokes, kholrabi, leeks, mushrooms, onions, parsnips, peas, spinach, swede (rutabaga) and turnips.

Jerusalem artichokes, potatoes, pumpkin and marrow

(squash), salsify, sweetcorn (corn), sweet potatoes and yams are classed as carbohydrates.

Salad foods

These include avocado, chicory (Belgian endive), cress, cucumber, garlic, lettuce (all types), olives, (bell) peppers, radishes, spring onions (scallions), bean sprouts and sprouted seeds, fresh, raw tomatoes and watercress.

TIPS

◆ Dressings for salads to be eaten with protein meals should be made from oil, cream, herbs and lemon or lime juice.

◆ Dressings for salads to be eaten with carbohydrate meals should be made from cream, soured (dairy sour) cream, olive oil or fresh tomato juice.

◆ Ready-made mayonnaise or salad cream is not recommended (see Russian Deluxe Salad page 110 for a home-made recipe).

Herbs and spices

These include all herbs, fresh or dried, all spices including the different peppercorns, curry powder and sweet spices such as cinnamon and nutmeg. Also included are organically grown grated citrus fruit rind, vanilla pod (bean) or natural vanilla essence (extract), yeast extract and vegetable stock cubes.

Nuts and seeds

Hazelnuts, walnuts, coconut, almonds, and poppy, pumpkin, sunflower and sesame seeds, for example.

Peanuts are not recommended.

Egg yolk

Raw egg white is not recommended.

Cooked whole eggs are part of the protein group.

Herb teas

Tea, coffee and cocoa are not recommended. If you must

drink tea or coffee, choose decaffeinated and drink with cream.

Setting agents

For example gelatine, vegetarian gelatines such as agar-agar (powdered seaweed) and Vege-Jel.

Foods To Avoid

- ❦ Fruits: cranberries, plums, rhubarb and stewed fresh fruit.
- ❦ Pulses: dried peas, beans and lentils and peanuts.
  Vegetarians use sparingly with neutral foods only.
- ❦ Pork and pork products such as ham, bacon and sausages.
- ❦ Processed fats, for example margarine and other 'bread spreads'.
- ❦ Raw egg white.
- ❦ Raw meat.
- ❦ Ready-made mayonnaise.
- ❦ Refined flour products, for example white flour, sweet and savoury biscuits, cakes and pasta made with white flour.
- ❦ Refined white rice.
- ❦ Smoked and cured products.
- ❦ Sugar and sugar products, for example refined sugars, syrups, jams, marmalade, ready-made meals and glucose.
- ❦ Tea, coffee, cocoa (see Herb Teas [page 17]).
- ❦ Vinegar. Use lemon or lime juice instead and only with protein-rich meals.

Watchpoints!

If you wish to lose weight you should use butter, oils and cream very sparingly indeed. Choose chicken, turkey or fish in preference to red meats and use semi-skimmed or skimmed milk and low-fat cheeses.

If you suffer from a kidney complaint you should avoid consuming large quantities of spinach, chestnuts, horseradish, mustard and pepper.

Watch your salt consumption. Too much salt is bad for you. Some cheeses and ready-made meals are high in salt and are therefore best avoided or eaten only in small quantities.

GETTING STARTED

Before starting food combining, it's a good idea to have a day of cleansing. That sounds daunting but it needn't be. Choose a day when you don't have much to do. Eat just fresh fruits and/or salad in any quantity whenever you feel peckish, and drink plenty of mineral water.

A Typical Day

The rest of this book is crammed with sumptuous breakfast, main meal, light meal and snack ideas for you to enjoy. But you don't always want to cook special recipes. Here's a suggested day's eating so you get an idea of what you can do just combining foods from the lists on pages 12–18 in the appropriate way. Quantities are up to you and your appetite. If you aren't a breakfast person, have a light meal of fruit and yoghurt or milk. Then have a neutral or protein lunch and a carbohydrate dinner.

First thing in the morning

A glass (about 250 ml/8 fl oz/1 cup) of hot or cold mineral water with a slice of lemon

Breakfast

Choose either a carbohydrate or a protein breakfast

Simple carbohydrate breakfast
Bowl of wholegrain cereal (such as Shredded Wheat) with a little buttermilk (NOT ordinary milk) or single (light) cream thinned with water
OR
Wholemeal bread, rolls or crispbread, spread with a little butter and honey
1 banana
Cup of herb tea

Simple protein breakfast
1 glass of pure orange or grapefruit juice
Eggs (maximum 2), cooked any way you like
Button mushrooms grilled or poached in a little water
Grilled tomato

Mid-morning snack

It's best to choose a protein snack in the morning and a carbohydrate snack in the afternoon. Try not to eat acid fruit after 3 pm as it is not so easy to digest.

Cup of herb tea or a glass of mineral water
and
1 piece of acid or stone fruit from the protein group (orange, apple, peach, etc)

Lunch

You can choose a neutral, a protein-rich or a carbohydrate-rich meal. Choose the opposite to breakfast or a neutral meal. But if you choose to have, say a protein-rich breakfast and a neutral lunch, you should have a carbohydrate-rich dinner in the evening.

Simple protein-rich lunch
Grated cheese and a mixed salad, dressed with a little olive oil, lemon juice and pepper
Fromage frais with a handful of fresh strawberries, raspberries or sliced stone fruit

Simple carbohydrate-rich lunch
Large baked jacket potato topped with soured (dairy sour) cream and chives and a mixed salad, dressed with fresh tomato juice whisked with a little olive oil and some black pepper
Fresh or dried figs

Simple neutral lunch
Basic mixed vegetable soup – any quantity of diced vegetables from the neutral group simmered in water with a vegetable stock cube and a bouquet garni sachet until tender
Piece of coconut

Mid-afternoon carbohydrate-rich snack
A cup of herbal tea
and
Slice of wholemeal bread and a scraping of butter

Dinner
Select the type of meal you have not yet had, so you end up with one protein-rich, one neutral and one carbohydrate-rich meal during the day.

Simple carbohydrate-rich dinner
Wholemeal pasta tossed with garlic, butter and chopped fresh herbs
A large mixed salad
A sweet, ripe pear, topped with crème fraîche and some chopped nuts

Simple protein-rich dinner
Grilled, lean sirloin steak
Grilled mushrooms, tomato and peas
A green salad dressed with a little olive oil, lemon juice and black pepper
Strawberries with or without cream

Simple neutral dinner
Mushrooms in garlic butter
Large mixed salad including avocado, olives and pine nuts, dressed with fresh tomato juice, blended with a little olive oil and freshly ground black pepper

Last thing at night
Glass of hot or cold mineral water with a slice of lemon

Four Weeks' Menus

This four-week cycle is intended just as a guide or to help you get used to balancing your meals. You can rearrange the days or meals on any one day to suit your lifestyle. Mix 'n' match as you please, making sure you get a neutral, a protein-rich and a carbohydrate-rich meal every day. I've suggested a whole range of afternoon snacks you can bake. Of course, you will probably want to make one at a time and have them each day until they're finished, then make a different one. (Or you could, for instance, make a Banana Tea Bread, cut into slices and freeze separately. Then you can take out a slice on whatever day you fancy it.) I haven't included the drinks. Drink plenty of mineral water through the day and have herbal tea (or decaffeinated tea or coffee occasionally) as you wish. Try to drink after meals or between them rather than with them if you can. If not, just sip your drink when you've thoroughly chewed and swallowed your mouthful.

Day 1

Protein-rich breakfast
½ grapefruit
Creamy Scrambled Eggs with Mushrooms (page 37)

Mid-morning snack
1 apple

Neutral lunch
Mediterranean Style Grilled Mixed Peppers (page 100)
Mixed Green Salad (page 123)

Mid-afternoon snack
Slice of Banana Tea Bread (page 131) and a scraping of butter

Carbohydrate-rich dinner
Spinach and Cashew Nut Parcels (page 88)
Tomato, Chive and Carrot Salad (page 124)
Fried Fruity Sandwich (page 149)

Day 2

Carbohydrate-rich breakfast
Porridge with Cream (page 48)
Wholemeal toast, a scraping of butter and yeast extract

Mid-morning snack
1 nectarine

Protein-rich lunch
Cheese Soufflé Omelette (page 71)
Tomato and Onion Salad (page 123)
Plain yoghurt

Mid-afternoon snack
Fruit Scone (page 132) with a scraping of butter

Neutral dinner
Creamy Baked Garlic Mushrooms (page 66)
Avocado and Bean Sprout Salad (page 125)
Spiced Almonds (page 155)

Day 3

Protein-rich breakfast
Glass of fresh orange juice
Devilled Kidneys (page 41)

Mid-morning snack
Slice of melon

Neutral lunch
Minted Cucumber and Soured Cream Dip with Crudités (page 67)
Tangy Chestnut Kebabs (page 100)

Mid-afternoon snack
Cucumber and Cress Butter Sandwich (page 133)

Carbohydrate-rich dinner
Root Vegetable Pastie with Creamed Mushroom Sauce (page 90)
Mixed Green Salad (page 123)
Dried Fruit Compote (page 149)

Day 4

Carbohydrate-rich breakfast
Banana Buttermilk Shake (page 58)
Fruity Flapjacks (page 49)

Mid-morning snack
Apple and a finger of Cheddar cheese

Neutral lunch
Curried Parsnip Soup (page 63)
Carrot, Beetroot and Celeriac Salad (page 125)

Mid-afternoon snack
Slice of wholemeal bread and a scraping of butter

Protein-rich dinner
Sherried Chicken Casserole (page 75)
Buttered Onion Spinach (page 114)
Spiced Oranges (page 144)

Day 5

Protein-rich breakfast
½ grapefruit
Mumbled Eggs (page 38)

Mid-morning snack
1 plain yoghurt

Carbohydrate-rich lunch
Spiced Bulgar With Pine Nuts (page 87)
Date Slice (page 150)

Mid-afternoon snack
1 banana

Neutral dinner
Globe Artichoke with Herb Butter (page 70)
Warm Courgette and Carrot Salad (page 120)

Day 6

Carbohydrate-rich breakfast
Tropical Muesli (page 49) with buttermilk

Mid-morning snack
1 apple

Neutral lunch
Chilled Cucumber Soup (page 60)
Fennel and Hazelnut Crunch (page 121)

Mid-afternoon snack
Slice of wholemeal toast and a scraping of butter

Protein-rich dinner
Salmon with Spring Vegetables (page 73)
Zabaglione (page 143)

Day 7

Protein-rich breakfast
Mixed Fruit Platter with Quark (page 44)

Mid-morning snack
Finger of Edam cheese and carrot sticks

Carbohydrate-rich lunch
Country Vegetable Broth (page 86)
Chewy Apricot Bar (page 136)

Mid-afternoon snack
Jumbo Digestive Biscuit (page 137)

Neutral dinner
Russian Salad Deluxe (page 110)

Day 8

Carbohydrate-rich breakfast
Wholemeal Raisin Muffin (page 52) with a scraping of butter

Mid-morning snack
1 apple

Neutral lunch
Curried Vegetables with Coconut (page 99)

Mid-afternoon snack
Singin' Hinny (page 138)

Protein-rich dinner
Marinated Tofu Salad (page 77)
Peach Melba (page 146)

Day 9

Protein-rich breakfast
Citrus Cocktail (page 46)
Grilled Halloumi Cheese with Mushrooms (page 43)

Mid-morning snack
Fruity Yoghurt Shake (page 127)

Neutral lunch
Asparagus with Green Hollandaise (page 69)
Italian Salad (page 126)

Mid-afternoon snack
2 Dropped Scones (page 139)

Carbohydrate-rich dinner
Vegetable Risotto (page 89)
Branflake Cake (page 142)

Day 10

Carbohydrate-rich breakfast
Stewed Figs (page 57)
Oatcakes (page 54) with a scraping of butter

Mid-morning snack
1 apple

Protein-rich lunch
Chicken and Vegetable Stir-fry (page 76)
Pineapple with Coconut (page 146)

Mid-Afternoon snack
Vitality Scone (page 141)

Neutral dinner
French Onion Soup (page 34)
Avocado Salad with Rosy Dressing (page 106)

Day 11

Protein-rich breakfast
1 glass of grapefruit juice
Baked Eggs in Tomatoes (page 38)

Mid-morning snack
Cheese-stuffed Celery (page 128)

Carbohydrate-rich lunch
Pasta with Green Beans and Basil (page 92)
Spiced Honey Toasts (page 152)

Mid-afternoon snack
2–4 fresh dates

Neutral dinner
Vegetable Terrine (page 105)
Mixed Green Salad (page 123)

Day 12

Carbohydrate-rich breakfast
Savoury Mushroom Toasts (page 55)

Mid-morning snack
Tomato Pick-me-up (page 130)

Neutral lunch
Bortsch with Soured Cream (page 61)
Dry-roasted Nuts (page 156)

Mid-afternoon snack
Italian Open Sandwich (page 132)

Protein-rich dinner
Trout with Almonds and Herbs (page 74)
Celery and Carrot Pot (page 115)
Strawberry Yoghurt Brûlé (page 144)

Day 13

Protein-rich breakfast
Peach and Cottage Cheese Pleasure (page 43)

Mid-morning snack
1 apple

Neutral lunch
Fresh Tomato Juice (page 64)
Carrot and Swede Cream with Crudités (page 67)

Mid-afternoon snack
Peanut Butter and Cress Pinwheel (page 134)

Carbohydrate-rich dinner
Vegetable Fajitas (page 94)
Chilli Salsa (page 94)
Butterscotch Bananas (page 152)

Day 14

Carbohydrate-rich breakfast
Honey Nut Oats (page 50)

Mid-morning snack
Fresh Strawberry Milkshake (page 127)

Protein-rich lunch
Beef Stroganoff (page 82)
Broccoli and Cauliflower Stir-fry (page 115)
Fresh Blackberry and Apple Compote (page 147)

Mid-afternoon snack
Handful of nuts and raisins

Neutral dinner
Mushroom Pâté-stuffed Peppers (page 109)
Village Garden Salad (page 120)

Day 15

Protein-rich breakfast
Tropical Fruits with Raspberry and Yoghurt Sauce (page 45)

Mid-morning snack
Fennel-Cheese Boats (page 129)

Neutral lunch
Guacamole with Vegetable Dippers (page 64)
Blushing Buttermilk Shake (page 66)

Mid-afternoon snack
Slice of Banana Tea Bread (page 131) and a scraping of butter

Carbohydrate-rich dinner
Hot Potato Sauté (page 97)
Green Bean and Tomato Salad (page 124)
Pears with Rum and Raisin Sauce (page 151)

Day 16

Carbohydrate-rich breakfast
Oatmeal Bannocks (page 51) with a scraping of butter and honey

Mid-morning snack
1 or 2 clementines

Protein-rich lunch
Grilled Sirloin Steak Sorrento (page 83)
Puréed Carrots and Peas (page 116)
Lemon Velvet (page 145)

Mid-afternoon snack
Tomato and Chive Sandwich (page 134)

Neutral dinner
Spinach and Broad Bean Soup (page 62)
Poor Man's Caviare with Vegetable Dippers (page 65)

Day 17

Protein-rich breakfast
Glass of orange juice
Grilled Fresh Sardines and Tomatoes (page 40)

Mid-morning snack
1 apple

Neutral lunch
Shredded Vegetable Platter with Soured Cream Dressing (page 112)
Sweet Spiced Cashew Nuts (page 155)

Mid-afternoon snack
Slice of Carrot Cake (page 139)

Carbohydrate-rich dinner
Rotelli with Broccoli and Cream (page 91)
Peasant Mixed Salad (page 119)
Carob Chew (page 140)

Day 18

Carbohydrate-rich breakfast
Golden Flecked Porridge (page 48)

Mid-morning snack
Blackcurrant Cooler (page 129)

Protein-rich lunch
Braised Duck with Peas and Lettuce (page 84)
Nutty Cauliflower (page 116)
Mixed Berries with Crème Fraîche (page 145)

Mid-afternoon snack
Handful of raisins

Neutral dinner
Vegetable Consommé Julienne (page 63)
Nutty Slaw (page 121)

Day 19

Protein-rich breakfast
Glass of pineapple juice
Poached Eggs on a Bed (page 39)

Mid-morning snack
1 orange

Neutral lunch
Mushroom and Courgette Kebabs (page 102)
Athena Salad (page 122)

Mid-afternoon snack
2 Dropped Scones (page 139)

Carbohydrate-rich dinner
Savoury Spinach Layer (page 93)
Creamy Rice Pudding (page 151)

Day 20

Carbohydrate-rich breakfast
Stewed Dried Pears with Raisins (page 58)
Wholemeal toast, a scraping of butter and yeast extract

Mid-morning snack
1 plain yoghurt

Protein-rich lunch
Lemon-glazed Lamb Cutlets (page 81)
Fruity Red Cabbage (page 117)
Green beans
Cider Syllabub (page 148)

Mid-afternoon snack
Wholegrain crispbread with a scraping of butter

Neutral dinner
Iced Tomato Soup (page 59)
Broccoli with Hazelnut Sauce (page 117)

Day 21

Protein-rich breakfast
Fresh Florida Cocktail (page 46)
Mushroom Omelette Wedges (page 40)

Mid-morning snack
Bunch of grapes

Neutral lunch
Gingered Vegetable Stir-fry (page 102)

Mid-afternoon snack
Slice of Teacup Cake (page 140)

Carbohydrate-rich dinner
Mexican Avocado Salad (page 98)
Banana Cheese (page 150)

Day 22

Carbohydrate-rich breakfast
Creamy Mustard Mushrooms on Toast (page 56)

Mid-morning snack
1 plain yoghurt

Protein-rich lunch
Normandy Pheasant (page 85)
Mixed Green Salad (page 123)
Fresh Orange Jelly (page 148)

Mid-afternoon snack
Salad Sandwich (page 135)

Neutral dinner
Metze Starter (page 68)
Vegetable Dolmas (page 103)

Day 23

Protein-rich breakfast
Orange and Pineapple Boat (page 47)
Grilled Tomatoes with Mozzarella (page 44)

Mid-morning snack
1 apple

Neutral lunch
Spiced Vegetable Casserole (page 104)
Cooling Cucumber (page 122)

Mid-afternoon snack
2 wholegrain crispbreads with a scraping of sesame butter

Carbohydrate-rich dinner
Mexican Rice (page 95)
Pear and Banana Crumble (page 153)

Day 24

Carbohydrate-rich breakfast
Currant Soda Bread (page 53) with a scraping of butter

Mid-morning snack
1–2 clementines

Protein-rich lunch
Moules Marinière (page 72)
Caesar Salad Special (page 78)

Mid-afternoon snack
Sweet dessert pear

Neutral dinner
Summer Salad Platter (page 111)
Avocado Delight (page 157)

Day 25

Protein-rich breakfast
Grilled Grapefruit (page 47)
2 boiled eggs

Mid-morning snack
Yoghurt with Crushed Berries (page 130)

Neutral lunch
Asparagus with Zest Butter (page 70)
Red Slaw with Walnuts (page 118)

Mid-afternoon snack
Cinnamon Toast (page 136)

Carbohydrate-rich dinner
Tagliatelle with Corn and Mushrooms (page 92)
Sweet Papaya Sundae (page 153)

Day 26

Carbohydrate-rich breakfast
Hot Fruity Oats (page 51)
Slice of wholemeal toast and a scraping of butter

Mid-morning snack
1 peach

Protein-rich lunch
Watercress Roulade (page 79)
Sesame Bean Sprout Salad (page 118)
Tropical Fruits with Raspberry and Yoghurt Sauce (page 45)

Mid-afternoon snack
Cucumber and Mascarpone Sandwich (page 135)

Neutral dinner
Turkish Aubergine Slippers (page 107)
Mixed Leaf Salad (page 126)
Tropical Cool (page 157)

Day 27

Protein-rich breakfast
Glass of orange juice
Grilled Herring with Lemon (page 42)

Mid-morning snack
Vanilla Yoghurt Shake (page 128)

Neutral lunch
Spinach Mousse (page 109)
Rainbow Salad (page 119)

Mid-afternoon snack
Whole-rye crispbread with a scraping of butter and honey

Carbohydrate-rich dinner
Stuffed Cabbage with Cream Potatoes (page 96)
Crêpes with Maple Syrup (page 154)

Day 28

Carbohydrate-rich breakfast
Hash Browns (page 57)

Mid-morning snack
Fresh Apricot Yoghurt (page 128)

Neutral lunch
Clear Soup with Peas (page 60)
Root Vegetable Satay (page 101)

Mid-afternoon snack
Banana and Raisin Sandwich (page 133)

Protein-rich dinner
Fragrant Grilled Lamb with Tomatoes (page 80)
Braised Leeks (page 114)
Jaffa Apples (page 147)

NOTES ON THE RECIPES

❦ Ingredients are given in metric, imperial and American measures. Use only one set per recipe, do not interchange.

❦ All spoon measures are level:
    1 tsp = 5 ml
    1 tbsp = 15 ml

❦ Eggs are medium unless otherwise stated.

❦ Always wash fresh produce and peel where necessary before preparing according to the recipe. If possible use organically grown fruit and vegetables and free range meat and poultry.

❦ All herbs are fresh unless dried are specified. If substituting dried when fresh are called for, use only half the quantity (or less) as dried herbs are very pungent.

❦ All preparation and cooking times are approximate.

❦ Always cook in the centre of the oven unless otherwise stated and preheat the oven (if necessary) to the temperature specified in the recipe.

❦ To help you when looking for appropriate recipes, all protein-rich recipes are printed in one style, carbohydrate-rich in a second, and neutral in a third.

BREAKFASTS

PROTEIN-RICH

You can have any fresh fruit (except bananas and the other fruits from the carbohydrate group) plus any one of the following recipes. Cheese, yoghurt or plainly cooked eggs are fine too.

Creamy Scrambled Eggs with Mushrooms

SERVES 2

25 g/1 oz/2 tbsp butter
4-6 mushrooms, sliced
4 eggs, beaten
30 ml/2 tbsp single (light) cream
Salt and freshly ground black pepper

1 Melt the butter in a small non-stick saucepan.

2 Add the mushrooms and cook, stirring, for 2 minutes.

3 Add the eggs and cream and cook over a gentle heat, stirring all the time until scrambled but creamy. Remove from the heat. Season to taste and serve straight away.

Mumbled Eggs

SERVES 2

3 tomatoes, sliced
4 eggs
5 ml/1 tsp English mustard
Salt and freshly ground black pepper
15 ml/1 tbsp milk
50 g/2 oz/¼ cup low-fat soft cheese
10 ml/2 tsp single (light) cream

1 Arrange the tomato slices in a ring on two plates and warm under the grill (broiler).

2 Beat the eggs with the mustard and a little salt and pepper.

3 Put the milk and cheese in a small saucepan and heat, stirring until smooth.

4 Stir in the egg mixture and cook, over a low heat, stirring gently until just set.

5 Stir in the cream. Quickly spoon into the centres of the tomato rings and serve straight away.

Baked Eggs in Tomatoes

SERVES 2

2 beefsteak tomatoes
A little olive oil
2 large eggs
Freshly ground black pepper
25 g/1 oz/¼ cup Cheddar cheese, grated

1 Cut a slice off the rounded end of each tomato and scoop out the seeds.

2 Stand the tomato shells in lightly oiled individual dishes and brush inside and out with a little olive oil.

3 Carefully break an egg into each shell.

4 Season with pepper then cover with grated cheese.

5 Bake in a preheated oven at 180°C/350°F/gas mark 4 for 15 minutes for soft-cooked eggs, or 20 minutes for hard-cooked.

Poached Eggs on a Bed

SERVES 2

225 g/8 oz young spinach leaves
15 g/½ oz/1 tbsp butter
1 onion, sliced
50 g/2 oz button mushrooms, sliced
30 ml/2 tbsp soured (dairy sour) cream
Salt and freshly ground black pepper
2 or 4 eggs
15 ml/1 tbsp lemon juice

1 Wash the spinach in plenty of running water. Shake off the excess water, then tear into pieces and place in a non-stick saucepan. Cover and cook gently for 5 minutes, shaking the pan occasionally. Drain and chop the spinach then return to the saucepan.

2 Melt the butter in a frying pan (skillet) and fry (sauté) the onion for 2 minutes, stirring. Add the mushrooms and continue cooking, stirring, until tender. Add the onion, mushrooms and any cooking juices to the spinach. Stir well, add the cream and season to taste. Keep warm.

3 Fill the frying pan with water, add the lemon juice and bring just to the boil. Carefully break in the eggs and poach over a fairly low heat until cooked to your liking.

4 Divide the spinach mixture between two hot plates. Remove the eggs with a fish slice and slide on top of the spinach. Serve straight away.

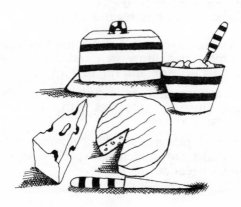

Mushroom Omelette Wedges

SERVES 2

75 g/3 oz button mushrooms, sliced
25 g/1 oz/2 tbsp butter
Good pinch of dried basil
Salt and freshly ground black pepper
4 eggs
30 ml/2 tbsp water
To garnish:
Sprigs of parsley

1 Cook the mushrooms in half the butter in an omelette pan until tender. Sprinkle with basil and a little salt and pepper.

2 Beat the eggs with the water.

3 Add the remaining butter to the pan and allow to sizzle. Pour in the egg mixture and cook, lifting and stirring until the mixture is just set.

4 Place the pan under a hot grill (broiler) until set and golden brown on top. Cut into four wedges and slide on to two warm plates. Garnish with parsley and serve.

Grilled Fresh Sardines and Tomatoes

SERVES 2

6 fresh sardines
Sunflower or olive oil
Coarse sea salt
2 ripe tomatoes, halved
5 ml/1 tsp chopped oregano

1 Cut off the sardine heads just behind the gills and squeeze out the intestines. Rinse well and dry on kitchen paper. Brush with a little oil and rub in a little sea salt.

2 Lay the fish on foil on a grill (broiler) rack with the tomatoes. Brush the tomatoes with oil and sprinkle with the oregano.

3 Cook under a hot grill for about 6 minutes, turning once, until the fish are golden and cooked through and the tomatoes are tender.

4 Serve straight away.

Devilled Kidneys

SERVES 2

4 lambs' kidneys
50 g/2 oz/¼ cup butter, softened
2.5 ml/½ tsp curry powder
1.5 ml/¼ tsp English mustard
2.5 ml/½ tsp paprika
15 ml/1 tbsp tomato purée (paste)
Salt and freshly ground black pepper

1 Remove any skin from the kidneys. Cut in halves lengthways and snip out the cores with scissors.

2 Thread on kebab skewers. Lay on foil on a grill (broiler) rack and dot with half the butter.

3 Mash the remaining butter with the flavourings, adding just a little salt and pepper.

4 Grill (broil) the kidneys for 3 minutes on each side, brushing with the melted butter on the grill rack.

5 Spread the flavoured butter over and return to the grill for 1 minute until bubbling. Serve piping hot.

TIP: If you like raw mushrooms, use a few to mop up the buttery juices.

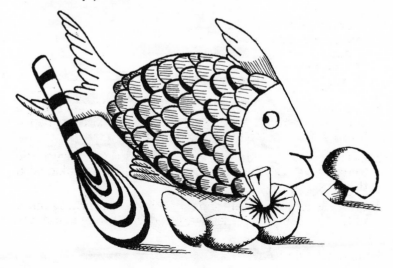

Grilled Herring with Lemon

SERVES 2

2 herrings, cleaned
Sunflower oil
30 ml/2 tbsp sesame seeds
10 ml/2 tsp lemon juice
Freshly ground black pepper
To garnish:
Lemon wedges
Sprigs of parsley

1 Carefully open out the herrings, skin sides up. Run your thumb up and down the backbones to loosen them then turn the fish over and carefully lift out the backbones. Remove any loose bones as well.

2 Brush very lightly with oil and place on a grill (broiler) rack.

3 Cook under a very hot grill for 3 minutes. Sprinkle with the sesame seeds, lemon juice and pepper and continue grilling for about 5 minutes until the fish are golden brown and cooked through.

4 Serve hot, garnished with lemon wedges and sprigs of parsley.

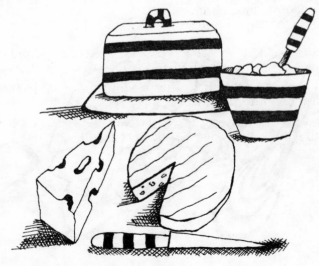

Grilled Halloumi Cheese with Mushrooms

SERVES 2

100 g/4 oz Halloumi cheese, cut in 4 slices
10 ml/2 tsp olive or sunflower oil
4 large, flat mushrooms
Freshly ground black pepper

1 Lay the cheese on a piece of foil on the grill (broiler) rack and brush both sides with a little of the oil.

2 Peel the mushrooms and place on the foil. Brush with the remaining oil and season well with freshly ground black pepper.

3 Grill (broil) for about 4 minutes, turning once, until the cheese is turning golden and the mushrooms are just cooked but still with some 'bite'. Put the cheese on the mushrooms and serve straight away.

Peach and Cottage Cheese Pleasure

SERVES 2

2 ripe peaches
100 g/4 oz/½ cup cottage cheese
Grated rind of ½ orange and the segments of
**   1 whole one, chopped**
60 ml/4 tbsp sesame seeds

1 Cut the peaches in halves, remove the stones and put two halves of peach on each of two shallow individual dishes.

2 Mix the cottage cheese with the orange rind and segments and spoon into the cavities of each peach half.

3 Toast the sesame seeds in a dry frying pan (skillet), stirring until golden. Sprinkle over the cheese and serve.

Grilled Tomatoes with Mozzarella

SERVES 2

4 ripe tomatoes, sliced
100 g/4 oz Mozzarella, thinly sliced
6–8 fresh basil leaves
10 ml/2 tsp olive oil

1 Arrange the tomato slices in a single layer on two flameproof plates.

2 Top with Mozzarella slices then scatter the basil over.

3 Drizzle with the oil then place under a hot grill (broiler) until the cheese melts and bubbles. Serve immediately.

Mixed Fruit Platter with Quark

SERVES 2

1 star fruit
1 mango
1 clementine
Handful of strawberries or cherries
1 kiwi fruit
150 ml/¼ pt/⅔ cup quark
10 ml/2 tsp chopped mint
To garnish:
Sprig of mint

1 Cut the star fruit across into four slices.

2 Peel the mango and cut the fruit off in neat slices round the stone.

3 Peel the clementine, remove as much pith as possible and separate into segments.

4 Hull and halve the strawberries or stone the cherries.

5 Peel and slice the kiwi fruit.

6 Arrange the fruits attractively on two serving plates.

7 Mix the quark with the chopped mint. Spoon to one side of the fruit and garnish with a sprig of mint before serving.

Tropical Fruits with Raspberry and Yoghurt Sauce

SERVES 2

1 avocado
Lemon juice
1 mango
10 lychees
175 g/6 oz raspberries
150 ml/¼ pt thick plain yoghurt
15–30 ml/1–2 tbsp apple juice

1 Peel, halve and stone the avocado. Cut into slices and dip in lemon juice to prevent discolouring.

2 Peel the mango and cut the fruit off the stone in neat slices.

3 Peel the lychees, cut in halves and remove the stones.

4 Purée the raspberries in a blender or food processor, then pass through a sieve (strainer) to remove the seeds.

5 Mix with the yoghurt. Sweeten and thin with the apple juice to taste.

6 Arrange the fruits attractively on two plates and drizzle the sauce over.

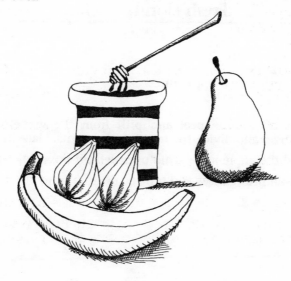

Citrus Cocktail

SERVES 2

1 pink grapefruit
1 orange
1 lime
45 ml/3 tbsp pineapple juice

1 Halve the grapefruit. Cut all round the fruit between the pith and the flesh then separate the fruit between each membrane. Lift out the fruit and place in a bowl then remove and discard the membranes (squeezing any juice over the fruit).

2 Cut off all the peel and pith from the orange (over the bowl with the grapefruit to catch any juice). Then cut the fruit into segments between each membrane and add to the grapefruit. Again, squeeze the membranes over the bowl to catch any last juice.

3 Grate the rind from the lime and add to the bowl. Squeeze the juice from the lime and mix with the pineapple juice. Add to the bowl and mix well. Pile back in the grapefruit skins in suitable dishes and spoon the juice over. Serve.

Fresh Florida Cocktail

SERVES 2

1 grapefruit
2 oranges
60 ml/4 tbsp apple juice
2 fresh cherries

1 Cut off all the peel and pith from the grapefruit and oranges and divide the fruit into segments. Place in a bowl.

2 Add the apple juice. Chill overnight, if possible.

3 Spoon into glasses and top each with a fresh cherry.

Orange and Pineapple Boats

SERVES 2

1 small pineapple
2 oranges
10 ml/2 tsp desiccated (shredded) coconut

1 Cut the pineapple in half. Using a serrated–edged knife, cut all the fruit off the skin. Cut out any hard central core and discard. Chop the flesh and put in a bowl.

2 Remove all peel and pith from the oranges. Cut in slices then cut each slice in quarters. Add to the pineapple with any juice.

3 Mix together then pile back into the pineapple skins.

4 Dry-fry the coconut in a frying pan (skillet) until golden and scatter over. Serve.

Grilled Grapefruit

SERVES 2

1 grapefruit
2 small knobs of butter

1 Cut the grapefruit in half. Using a serrated–edged knife cut all round the fruit between the pith and the flesh then loosen each piece of fruit between the membranes.

2 Place on a grill (broiler) rack and dot with butter.

3 Grill (broil) until the top is bubbling and just turning golden. Serve hot.

CARBOHYDRATE-RICH

You can have any fruits from the carbohydrate group such as bananas, dates, figs etc, plus any of the following. Wholemeal toast with a scraping of butter and honey or yeast extract is fine too or any of the wholegrain breakfast cereals but NOT with ordinary milk. It must be half buttermilk or single (light) cream, half water.

Porridge with Cream

SERVES 2

100 g/4 oz/1 cup rolled oats
450 ml/¾ pt/2 cups water
200 ml/7 fl oz/scant 1 cup single (light) cream
Good pinch of salt
To serve:
Clear honey (optional)

1 Blend the rolled oats with half the water in a non-stick saucepan. Stir in the remaining water, half the cream and the salt.

2 Bring to the boil, stirring all the time, and simmer for 5 minutes, stirring until creamy and thickened.

3 Turn into bowls and drizzle with the remaining cream and honey, if liked.

Variation: Golden Flecked Porridge
Prepare as for Porridge with Cream but stir in 75 g/3 oz/½ cup chopped sultanas (golden raisins) when cooking the porridge.

Fruity Flapjacks

MAKES 8

50 g/2 oz/¼ cup butter
60 ml/4 tbsp thick honey
175 g/6 oz/1½ cups rolled oats
50 g/2 oz/⅓ cup mixed dried fruit

1 Melt the butter and honey in a saucepan.

2 Stir in the oats then the fruit.

3 Turn into a greased 18 cm/7 in square baking tin (pan) and bake in a preheated oven at 180°C/350°F/gas mark 4 for about 20–25 minutes or until turning golden.

4 Leave to cool in the tin for 5 minutes, mark into fingers and leave to cool completely before removing. Store in an airtight tin.

Tropical Muesli

MAKES ABOUT 6 SERVINGS

225 g/8 oz/2 cups rolled oats
50 g/2 oz/⅓ cup dried pears, chopped
50 g/2 oz/⅓ cup dried banana slices
50 g/2 oz/½ cup coconut flakes
50 g/2 oz/½ cup chopped mixed nuts
50 g/2 oz/⅓ cup sultanas (golden raisins)
To serve:
Buttermilk, thinned with water, if liked

Mix all the ingredients together and serve with buttermilk. Store any unused mixture in an airtight container.

Hot Fruity Oats

SERVES 2–3

600 ml/1 pt/2½ cups water
65 g/2½ oz/good ½ cup medium oatmeal
50 g/2 oz/⅓ cup chopped dates
50 g/2 oz/⅓ cup sultanas (golden raisins)
50 g/2 oz/⅓ cup currants
To serve:
Single (light) cream

1 Put the water in a heavy-based saucepan. Bring to the boil.

2 Pour in the oatmeal in a steady stream, stirring constantly. Bring back to the boil.

3 Reduce the heat as low as possible, cover and cook very gently for 10 minutes, stirring occasionally.

4 Stir in the fruits and continue cooking for a further 10 minutes until really creamy.

5 Spoon into bowls and serve with a little cream.

Honey Nut Oats

MAKES ABOUT 12 SERVINGS

100 g/4 oz/1 cup sesame seeds
225 g/8 oz/2 cups rolled oats
225 g/8 oz/2 cups hazelnuts, roughly chopped
100 g/4 oz/1 cup sunflower seeds
90 ml/6 tbsp clear honey
60 ml/4 tbsp hand-hot water
50 g/2 oz/¼ cup butter
100 g/4 oz/⅔ cup raisins
To serve (optional):
Single (light) cream blended with an equal quantity
of water

1 Toast the sesame seeds in a dry frying pan (skillet) until golden then tip into a large bowl.

2 Add the oats, nuts and sunflower seeds and mix well.

3 Blend the honey with the water and stir into the dry mixture with the melted butter.

4 When well mixed turn into a lightly oiled baking tin (pan) and spread evenly.

5 Bake in a preheated oven at 160°C/325°F/gas mark 3 for about 1 hour, stirring from time to time until crisp, golden and crumbly.

6 Stir in the raisins and leave to cool. Store in an airtight tin and serve plain or with the single cream blended with water.

Oatmeal Bannocks

MAKES 6

175 g/6 oz/1½ cups wholemeal flour
15 ml/1 tbsp baking powder
2.5 ml/½ tsp salt
50 g/2 oz/½ cup fine oatmeal
25 g/1 oz/2 tbsp butter
15 ml/1 tbsp clear honey
150 ml/¼ pt/⅔ cup water

1 Mix the flour, baking powder, salt and oatmeal together in a bowl.

2 Rub in the butter then stir in the honey and mix with enough water to form a soft but not sticky dough.

3 Knead gently on a lightly floured surface, pat out to a rectangle about 1 cm/½ in thick and cut into six square cakes.

4 Cook in a hot non-stick frying pan (skillet) for about 5 minutes until golden brown underneath, then turn over and cook for 5 minutes more until golden and well risen.

5 Serve warm, split and lightly spread with butter and honey.

Wholemeal Raisin Muffins

MAKES 12

450g/1 lb wholemeal flour
5 ml/1 tsp salt
1 sachet easy-blend dried yeast
25 g/1 oz/2 tbsp butter
300 ml/½ pt/1¼ cups water
150 ml/¼ pt/⅔ cup buttermilk
75 g/3 oz/½ cup raisins
A little extra wholemeal flour for dusting

1 Mix the flour, salt and yeast in a bowl.

2 Melt the butter in a saucepan and add the water and buttermilk. Heat to hand-hot.

3 Pour into the flour mixture, add the raisins and beat with a wooden spoon until smooth and elastic (the mixture will be too wet to knead).

4 Cover the bowl with oiled cling film (plastic wrap) and leave in a warm place until the mixture doubles in bulk (about 1 hour).

5 Knock back the dough then divide into 12 pieces. With flour-coated hands, shape the pieces into balls, place well apart on a well-floured baking sheet and flatten slightly. Cover with oiled cling film and leave in a warm place for 45 minutes to rise.

6 Heat a lightly greased heavy-based frying pan (skillet) and carefully transfer four muffins to the pan. Cook over a low heat for 8–10 minutes on each side until golden and cooked through. Repeat with the remaining mixture.

7 Serve warm with a scraping of butter.

TIP: Muffins are wonderful freshly cooked but you can make them in advance, then warm in the microwave or a slow oven, or pull apart and toast under a hot grill (broiler).

Currant Soda Bread

MAKES 1 LOAF

450 g/1 lb wholemeal flour
10 ml/2 tsp bicarbonate of soda (baking soda)
10 ml/2 tsp cream of tartar
5 ml/1 tsp mixed (apple pie) spice
25 g/1 oz/2 tbsp butter
100 g/4 oz/⅔ cup currants
300 ml/½ pt/1¼ cups buttermilk

1 Mix the dry ingredients in a bowl.

2 Rub in the butter and stir in the currants.

3 Mix with the buttermilk to form a soft but not sticky dough.

4 Shape into a ball on a lightly floured surface and transfer to a baking sheet. Flatten slightly and mark in quarters with the back of a knife.

5 Bake in a preheated oven at 220°C/425°F/gas mark 7 for about 25 minutes until risen, golden and the base sounds hollow when tapped. Leave to cool on a wire rack.

6 Break into quarters then slice thickly and serve with a scraping of butter.

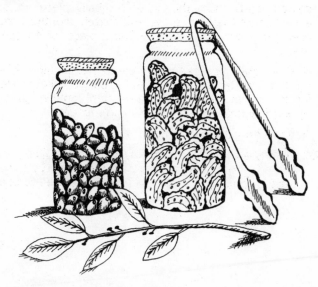

Oatcakes

MAKES 8

75g/3 oz/¾ cup medium oatmeal
Good pinch of salt
1.5 ml/¼ tsp bicarbonate of soda (baking soda)
15 g/½ oz/1 tbsp butter, melted
60 ml/4 tbsp hand-hot water
A little extra oatmeal for dusting
Sunflower oil for greasing

1 Mix all the ingredients except the oil together in a bowl until the mixture forms a dough.

2 Turn out on to a surface dusted with oatmeal and roll out thinly to a large round about 25 cm/10 in.

3 Cut into eight wedges.

4 Lightly oil a large frying pan (skillet) and cook the oatcakes a few at a time until firm. Carefully turn them over so they don't break and cook the other sides for 2 minutes more. Cool on a wire rack.

5 Serve with a scraping of butter. Store in an airtight container.

Savoury Mushroom Toasts

SERVES 2

100 g/4 oz button mushrooms
15 g/½ oz/1 tbsp butter
15 ml/1 tbsp water
1.5 ml/¼ tsp paprika
Freshly ground black pepper
2 slices wholemeal bread
A little extra butter
Yeast extract
To garnish:
Chopped parsley

1 Put the mushrooms in a pan with the butter and water. Cover and cook for 3 minutes, shaking the pan occasionally.

2 Remove the lid, add the paprika and lots of black pepper. Boil rapidly, stirring until any liquid has evaporated.

3 Toast the bread on both sides and spread with a little butter and yeast extract. Transfer to warm plates.

4 Spoon the mushrooms on top and serve garnished with chopped parsley.

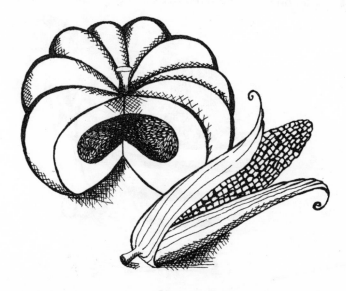

Creamy Mustard Mushrooms on Toast

SERVES 2

1 small onion, chopped
15 g/½ oz butter
100 g/4 oz button mushrooms
5 ml/1 tsp English mustard
7.5 ml/1½ tsp cornflour (cornstarch)
150 ml/¼ pt/⅔ cup soured (dairy sour) cream
Salt and freshly ground black pepper
To serve:
2 slices wholemeal toast, lightly buttered
To garnish:
Cayenne

1 Fry (sauté) the onion in the butter for 2 minutes, stirring until softened but not browned.

2 Add the mushrooms and continue cooking for 4–5 minutes until tender and the liquid has been absorbed.

3 Blend the mustard and cornflour with the cream and stir into the mushrooms. Season well. Simmer for a further 3 minutes, stirring until thickened.

4 Spoon on to hot buttered toast and garnish with cayenne.

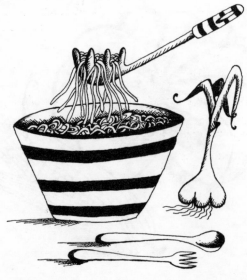

Hash Browns

SERVES 2

2 large potatoes, diced
15 ml/1 tbsp sunflower oil
1 onion, finely chopped
2.5 ml/½ tsp paprika
Salt and freshly ground black pepper
To serve:
Cherry tomatoes (optional)

1 Cook the potatoes in boiling, lightly salted water for about 5 minutes or until tender. Drain.

2 Meanwhile, heat the oil in a frying pan (skillet) and fry (sauté) the onion for 2 minutes, stirring.

3 Add the potatoes, paprika and a little salt and pepper and fry, tossing over a high heat until golden brown and the potatoes are starting to break up.

4 Press down firmly with a fish slice and cook without disturbing for a further 2–3 minutes. Divide in half and serve straight from the pan with fresh cherry tomatoes, if liked.

Stewed Figs

SERVES 4

8 fresh figs
300 ml/½ pt/1¼ cups water
10 ml/2 tsp honey or to taste

1 Place the figs in a saucepan with the water and honey.

2 Bring to the boil, cover, reduce the heat and simmer for 5–10 minutes until really tender.

3 Taste and add more honey if liked. Leave to cool then chill before serving.

Stewed Dried Pears with Raisins

SERVES 2–4

225 g/8 oz dried pears
75 g/3 oz/½ cup raisins
300 ml/½ pt/1¼ cups cold decaffeinated tea
Honey to taste

1 Soak the pears and raisins in the cold tea for at least 2 hours but preferably overnight.

2 Bring to the boil, reduce the heat, cover and simmer very gently for about 20 minutes until the pears are very soft. Leave to cool.

3 Sweeten with honey if necessary, then chill before serving.

Banana Buttermilk Shake

SERVES 1

1 ripe banana
200 ml/7 fl oz/scant 1 cup cold buttermilk
Pinch of ground cinnamon
Crushed ice

1 Purée the banana in a blender or food processor.

2 Add the buttermilk and cinnamon and run the machine until the mixture is blended and frothy.

3 Pour over crushed ice in a tall glass and serve straight away.

STARTERS AND LIGHT MEALS

These dishes are ideal for light lunches or suppers or can be served as starters for a more elaborate meal in which case serve smaller quantities. As they are all neutral they can be served before any main meal you like from a big, juicy steak to a steaming bowl of pasta. Turn any of the soups into carbohydrate meals by serving with wholemeal bread or rolls.

NEUTRAL

Iced Tomato Soup

SERVES 4

750 g/1½ lb ripe tomatoes, roughly chopped
15 ml/1 tbsp olive oil
45 ml/3 tbsp crème fraîche
2.5 ml/½ tsp English mustard
5 ml/1 tsp dried oregano
Salt and freshly ground black pepper
150 ml/¼ pt/⅔ cup cold vegetable stock
To garnish:
A little extra crème fraîche
Snipped chives

1 Purée the tomatoes in a blender or processor, then sieve (strain) into a bowl or jug.

2 Stir in the remaining ingredients and chill until ready to serve.

3 Pour into soup bowls and garnish each with a small spoonful of crème fraîche and a sprinkling of snipped chives.

Chilled Cucumber Soup

SERVES 4

1 cucumber
Salt
10 ml/2 tsp dried dill (dill weed)
Freshly ground black pepper
300 ml/½ pt/1¼ cups soured (dairy sour) cream
300 ml/½ pt/1¼ cups buttermilk, chilled

1 Cut four slices off the cucumber and reserve for garnish. Grate the remainder into a bowl.

2 Sprinkle with a little salt, stir and leave to stand for 10 minutes.

3 Stir in the dill, lots of pepper and the soured cream. Chill for at least an hour to allow the flavours to develop.

4 Stir in the cold buttermilk and thin with water if liked, ladle into soup bowls and garnish each with a reserved slice of cucumber.

Clear Soup with Peas

SERVES 2

750 ml/1¼ pts/3 cups water
2 vegetable stock cubes
1 carrot, cut into chunks
1 onion, halved
½ bay leaf
50 g/2 oz fresh, shelled or frozen peas
Salt and freshly ground black pepper

1 Put the water in a saucepan with the crumbled stock cubes, carrot, onion and bay leaf. Bring to the boil, reduce the heat, part-cover and simmer for 30 minutes.

2 Remove the carrot, onion and bay leaf with a draining spoon.

3 Add the peas and simmer, uncovered for 5 minutes or until tender. Season to taste.

4 Ladle into soup bowls and serve.

Bortsch with Soured Cream

SERVES 4

2 carrots, coarsely grated
2 celery sticks, grated
1 onion, grated
3 cooked beetroot (red beets), about 350 g/12 oz in
all, grated
900 ml/1½ pts/3¾ cups vegetable stock
Grated rind of ½ lemon
Salt and freshly ground black pepper
To serve:
150 ml/¼ pt/⅔ cup soured (dairy sour) cream
Paprika

1 Put all the grated vegetables in a large saucepan.

2 Add the stock, lemon rind and a little salt and pepper.

3 Bring to the boil, reduce the heat, part-cover and simmer for 20 minutes until the vegetables are really tender. Taste and re-season if necessary.

4 Ladle into warm soup bowls. Top each with a little soured cream and dust with paprika before serving.

French Onion Soup

SERVES 4

This is also delicious served as a protein-rich soup by sprinkling with grated Gruyère (Swiss) cheese before serving.

40g/1½ oz/3 tbsp butter
4 large onions, roughly chopped
1 litre/1¾ pts/4¼ cups vegetable stock
Salt and freshly ground black pepper

1 Melt the butter in a heavy-based saucepan.

2 Add the onions and fry (sauté), stirring for 10 minutes until the onions are a rich golden brown.

3 Stir in the stock, bring to the boil, reduce the heat, part-cover and simmer for 15 minutes until the onions are really soft. Season to taste and ladle into soup bowls.

Spinach and Broad Bean Soup

SERVES 4

1 onion, chopped
15 g/½ oz/1 tbsp butter
450 g/1 lb spinach
175 g/6 oz shelled broad (lima) beans
Good pinch of grated nutmeg
750 ml/1¼ pts/3 cups vegetable stock
Salt and freshly ground black pepper
150 ml/¼ pt/⅔ cup single (light) cream

1 Fry (sauté) the onion in the butter for 2 minutes, stirring.

2 Tear the spinach leaves into pieces, discarding any thick stalks and add to the pan. Cook, stirring for 1 minute until they start to soften.

3 Add the broad beans, nutmeg, stock and a little seasoning. Bring to the boil, reduce the heat, cover and simmer gently for 20 minutes or until the vegetables are very tender.

4 Purée in a blender or food processor and return to the saucepan. Stir in the cream, taste and re-season if necessary. Ladle into soup bowls and serve hot, or cool, chill and serve very cold.

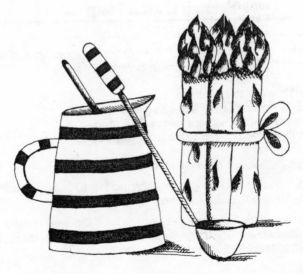

Vegetable Consommé Julienne

SERVES 2–3

1 carrot, cut into very thin matchsticks
1 turnip, cut into very thin matchsticks
¼ head of celeriac (celery root), cut into very thin matchsticks
750 ml/1¼ pts/3 cups water
2 vegetable stock cubes
5 ml/1 tsp yeast extract
Freshly ground black pepper

1 Put the prepared vegetables in a saucepan with the water and stock cubes.

2 Bring to the boil, reduce the heat and cook over a moderate heat for about 20 minutes until the vegetables are really tender.

3 Stir in the yeast extract and season to taste with pepper. Ladle into warm bowls and serve.

Curried Parsnip Soup

SERVES 4

450 g/1 lb parsnips, sliced
1 onion, chopped
25 g/1 oz/2 tbsp butter
15 ml/1 tbsp curry powder
600 ml/1 pt/2½ cups vegetable stock
300 ml/½ pt/1¼ cups single (light) cream
Salt and freshly ground black pepper
To garnish:
Chopped parsley

1 Put the parsnips, onion, butter and curry powder in a pan. Cook, stirring for 3 minutes.

2 Stir in the stock, bring to the boil, part cover and simmer for 15 minutes or until the parsnips are tender.

3 Purée in a blender or food processor then return to the saucepan.

4 Stir in the cream and season to taste. Heat through then serve garnished with chopped parsley.

Fresh Tomato Juice

SERVES 2–3

450 g/1 lb very ripe tomatoes
½ small onion
5 ml/1 tsp dried basil
Salt and freshly ground black pepper

1 Roughly cut up the tomatoes and place in a blender or food processor with the onion and basil.

2 Run the machine until smooth.

3 Sieve (strain) to remove the pips and little bits of skin.

4 Season to taste then chill until ready to serve.

Guacamole with Vegetable Dippers

SERVES 2

1 ripe avocado
1 fresh green chilli, seeded and chopped
Grated rind of ½ lemon
½ small garlic clove, crushed
30 ml/2 tbsp olive oil
Salt and freshly ground black pepper
2.5 cm/1 in piece of cucumber, finely chopped
1 tomato, finely chopped
1 each of red, green and yellow (bell) peppers,
**   cut into thickish strips**
2–3 courgettes (zucchini), cut into matchsticks

1 Peel and remove the stone from the avocado.

2 Mash in a bowl with the chilli, lemon rind and garlic.

3 Gradually work in the olive oil until smooth and creamy.

4 Season to taste and fold in the chopped cucumber and tomato.

5 Turn into two small pots and place on serving plates.

6 Arrange the peppers and courgettes around the pots of guacamole and serve.

Poor Man's Caviare with Vegetable Dippers

SERVES 2

1 aubergine (eggplant)
¼ small onion, very finely chopped
1 small garlic clove, crushed
2 tomatoes, skinned and finely chopped
45 ml/3 tbsp olive oil
Salt and freshly ground black pepper
To serve:
1 head of chicory (Belgian endive),
   separated into leaves
5 cm/2 in piece of cucumber, cut into matchsticks
½ small cauliflower, cut into tiny florets
12 button mushrooms
A handful of walnut halves

1 Cut the stalk off the aubergine then place under a hot grill (broiler) for about 20 minutes, turning a few times until the skin is blackened and the flesh feels soft.

2 Cool slightly then split and scoop out the flesh. Finely chop and place in a bowl. Discard the skin.

3 Add the onion, garlic and tomatoes and then gradually beat in the oil a little at a time. Season to taste.

4 Spoon into a serving bowl and arrange the 'dippers' around.

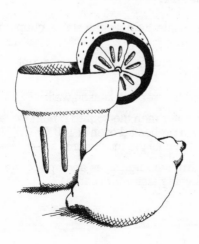

Blushing Buttermilk Shake

SERVES 1

2 cooked beetroot (red beets), roughly cut up
Pinch of paprika
75 ml/5 tbsp water
150 ml/¼ pt/⅔ cup buttermilk, chilled
Freshly ground black pepper

1 Purée the beetroot with the paprika in a blender or food processor.

2 Add the water and buttermilk and run the machine until smooth and frothy. Season to taste with pepper. Pour over ice cubes in a tall glass and serve immediately.

Creamy Baked Garlic Mushrooms

SERVES 2

8 large, flat mushrooms
15 g/½ oz/1 tbsp butter
1 small garlic clove, crushed
Salt and freshly ground black pepper
15 ml/1 tbsp water
150 ml/¼ pt/⅔ cup soured (dairy sour) cream
To garnish:
Chopped parsley

1 Peel the mushrooms. Remove the stalks, chop and scatter over the gills.

2 Use the butter to grease a shallow ovenproof dish then lay the mushrooms in it.

3 Sprinkle the garlic over and season well.

4 Pour over the water then the soured cream, cover with foil or a lid and bake in a preheated oven at 190°C/375°F/gas mark 5 for about 20 minutes until the mushrooms are cooked through.

5 Transfer to warm serving plates and spoon the creamy juices over. Sprinkle with parsley and serve.

Minted Cucumber and Soured Cream Dip with Crudités

SERVES 2

½ cucumber, grated
150 ml/¼ pt/⅔ cup soured (dairy sour) cream
1 small garlic clove, crushed (optional)
5 ml/1 tsp dried mint
Salt and freshly ground black pepper
To serve:
2 carrots, cut into matchsticks
2 celery sticks cut into matchsticks
12 radishes
1 green (bell) pepper, cut in strips

1 Squeeze the cucumber firmly to remove excess juices.

2 Place in a bowl and add the soured cream, garlic, if using, mint and a little salt and pepper. Chill until ready to serve.

3 Spoon into two small pots and place in the centre of two serving plates. Arrange the prepared vegetables around and serve.

Carrot and Swede Cream with Crudités

SERVES 4

1 small swede (rutabaga), diced
3 carrots, diced
100 g/4 oz/½ cup Mascarpone cheese
15 g/½ oz/1 tbsp butter
Salt and freshly ground black pepper
1.5 ml/¼ tsp cayenne
10 ml/2 tsp toasted sesame seeds
To serve:
Sticks of raw carrot, cucumber, celery,
    courgettes (zucchini) and red (bell) peppers

1 Boil the swede and carrots in lightly salted water until tender.

2 Drain and purée in a blender or food processor with the Mascarpone cheese and the butter.

3 Season to taste, spoon into two or three small pots and sprinkle with the sesame seeds.

4 Arrange the crudités around and serve warm.

Metze Starter

SERVES 2–4

This is a Greek Cypriot way of serving nibbles with drinks. Any suitable salad items can be used or any of the dips given in this section. Turn it into a protein meal by adding a bowl of diced Feta cheese and a couple of hard-boiled (hard-cooked) eggs.

Or make it a carbohydrate meal by adding a potato salad dressed with soured (dairy sour) cream or home-made mayonnaise (see Russian Deluxe Salad page 110)

2 cooked beetroot (red beets), diced
30 ml/2 tbsp soured (dairy sour) cream
15 ml/1 tbsp snipped chives
2 carrots, grated
15 ml/1 tbsp sesame seeds, toasted
2 green (bell) peppers, cut into large dice
15 ml/1 tbsp olive oil
Coarse sea salt
Handful of cherry tomatoes
¼ cucumber, diced
1 bunch of radishes

1 Mix the beetroot with the soured cream, place in a small bowl and sprinkle with the chives.

2 Put the carrots in a separate bowl and sprinkle with the sesame seeds.

3 Fry (sauté) the peppers in the oil, tossing until turning golden. Turn into a small bowl and sprinkle with sea salt.

4 Put the tomatoes, cucumber and radishes in three separate bowls.

5 Arrange on the table and serve.

Asparagus with Green Hollandaise

SERVES 2

350 g/12 oz asparagus
Sauce:
1 egg yolk
Grated rind of ½ large lemon
Freshly ground black pepper
Pinch of cayenne
50 g/2 oz/¼ cup butter, melted
½ bunch of watercress, chopped
15 ml/1 tbsp chopped parsley

1 Trim off about 5 cm/2 in from the base of the stems of asparagus and tie the spears in a bundle.

2 Stand the asparagus in a pan of lightly salted water. Cover with a lid (or foil if the spears are too tall for the pan).

3 Bring to the boil, reduce the heat and cook over a moderate heat for 10 minutes. Turn off the heat and leave for 5 minutes. Drain.

4 Meanwhile, whisk the egg yolk in a bowl with the lemon rind, some black pepper and the cayenne.

5 Gradually whisk in the melted butter.

6 Stand the bowl over a pan of gently simmering water and whisk until the mixture is thick and pale (about 5–10 minutes). Do not allow to boil or the mixture will curdle.

7 Stir in the watercress and parsley.

8 Lay the asparagus on two warm plates and spoon the sauce over just below the spear heads.

Asparagus with Zest Butter

SERVES 2

350 g/12 oz asparagus
50 g/2 oz/¼ cup butter
Grated rind of 1 orange
Grated rind of ½ lemon
10 ml/2 tsp snipped chives
Freshly ground black pepper

1 Prepare the asparagus as for Asparagus with Green Hollandaise (page 69).

2 Melt the butter with the orange and lemon rind and the chives. Sizzle for 2 minutes.

3 Arrange the asparagus on warm plates and drizzle the zest butter over. Serve straight away.

Globe Artichokes with Herb Butter

SERVES 2

2 globe artichokes
50 g/2 oz/¼ cup butter
15 ml/1 tbsp chopped parsley
15 ml/1 tbsp snipped chives
10 ml/2 tsp chopped basil

1 Twist off the artichoke stalks and trim the bases level so they will stand up.

2 Cook in boiling salted water for about 20 minutes or until a leaf pulls away easily. Remove from the pan with a draining spoon and drain upside down on kitchen paper.

3 Meanwhile melt the butter in a small saucepan and stir in the herbs. Pour into two little dishes and serve with the artichokes.

To eat: Pull off each leaf in turn and dip the base in the butter. Draw through the teeth to remove the fleshy part. Discard the leaf. Continue until all the leaves are eaten and the hairy choke is revealed. Cut this off and discard then eat the heart with a knife and fork, dipping it in any remaining herb butter.

Main Meals

All these meals are highly nutritious. Some of them may seem rather rich at first as you aren't having starch such as rice, pasta or potatoes to soak up sauces and so on. However, eating plenty of vegetables or salad with them makes them very digestible and you will come to enjoy the delicious flavours of the proteins unmasked by stodge. I prefer to eat protein-rich main meals at lunch-time when I can to allow plenty of time for them to digest properly but the choice is yours.

Cheese Soufflé Omelette

SERVES 1

2 eggs, separated
10 ml/2 tsp water
Salt and freshly ground black pepper
25 g/1 oz/¼ cup Cheddar cheese, grated
15 ml/1 tbsp butter

1 Beat the egg yolks with the water and a little salt and pepper. Stir in the cheese.

2 Whisk the egg whites and fold into the egg yolk mixture.

3 Heat the butter in a non-stick omelette pan. Add the egg mixture and cook over a gentle heat until setting underneath. Lift gently with a palette knife to check it is not getting too brown.

4 When the omelette is nicely browned, after about 3–4 minutes, place the pan under a hot grill (broiler) until the omelette puffs up and is golden on top. Serve immediately.

Moules Marinière

SERVES 2

1 kg/2¼ lb fresh mussels in their shells
25 g/1 oz/2 tbsp butter
1 small onion, finely chopped
1 wineglass white wine
1 wineglass water
Freshly ground black pepper
20 ml/4 tsp chopped parsley

1 Scrub the mussels, pull off the beards and scrape off any barnacles. Discard any that are broken or open and won't close immediately they are tapped. Rinse well.

2 Melt the butter in a large saucepan. Add the onion and fry (sauté) gently for 2 minutes until soft but not brown.

3 Add the mussels, the wine and water and a good grinding of pepper. Cover, bring to the boil and cook over a moderate heat for 5 minutes, shaking the pan occasionally.

4 Discard any mussels that have not opened. Stir in the parsley. Ladle into large soup bowls including all the juices and serve straight away.

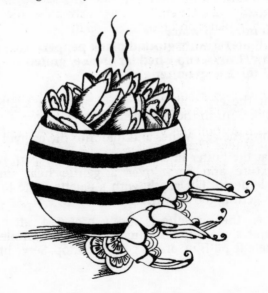

Salmon with Spring Vegetables

SERVES 2

2 salmon steaks (about 175 g/6 oz each)
Water
1 bay leaf
1 carrot, sliced
1 small onion, sliced
6 peppercorns
Butter Mayonnaise:
1 egg yolk
Good pinch each of dry mustard, salt and pepper
50 g/2 oz/¼ cup butter, melted
15 ml/1 tbsp lemon juice
75 ml/5 tbsp whipping cream, whipped
To serve:
100 g/4 oz mangetout (snow peas)
100 g/4 oz baby carrots
100 g/4 oz baby turnips
100 g/4 oz French beans

1 Put the fish in a shallow pan with the water, bay leaf, carrot, onion and peppercorns. Cover, bring to the boil then turn off the heat and leave the fish to stand until the water is cold. Carefully lift out with a fish slice. Transfer to serving plates and remove the skin.

2 Meanwhile, make the butter mayonnaise. Beat the egg yolk with the seasonings. Gradually whisk in the melted butter a drop at a time until thick and creamy.

3 Whisk in the lemon juice then fold in the whipped cream. Taste and re-season if necessary. Chill until ready to serve.

4 Steam or boil the vegetables in lightly salted water until just tender. Drain, rinse with cold water and drain again.

5 Arrange the vegetables around the fish attractively and serve with the mayonnaise.

Trout with Almonds and Herbs

SERVES 2

2 trout, cleaned
Salt and freshly ground black pepper
15 g/½ oz/1 tbsp butter
30 ml/2 tbsp flaked almonds
15 ml/1 tbsp sunflower oil
150 ml/¼ pt/⅔ cup soured (dairy sour) cream
15 ml/1 tbsp snipped chives
15 ml/1 tbsp chopped parsley
To serve:
Celery and Carrot Pot (see page 115)

1 Rinse the fish under cold running water and pat dry with kitchen paper. Season and remove the heads, if preferred.

2 Heat the butter in a frying pan (skillet) and fry (sauté) the almonds until lightly golden. Remove from the pan with a draining spoon.

3 Add the oil to the butter in the pan. Heat through then add the fish and fry for 3 minutes on each side to brown.

4 Add the soured cream, herbs and a little more seasoning, if liked. Cover with a lid or foil and cook for a further 6–8 minutes until the fish is cooked through.

5 Transfer to warm serving plates, spoon over the sauce then scatter with the almonds. Serve hot with Celery and Carrot Pot.

Sherried Chicken Casserole

SERVES 4

1 onion, sliced
2 carrots, thinly sliced
15 ml/1 tbsp olive oil
4 chicken portions
75 g/3 oz button mushrooms, halved
400 g/14 oz/1 large can chopped tomatoes
30 ml/2 tbsp sherry
Salt and freshly ground black pepper
1 bouquet garni sachet
To serve:
Buttered Onion Spinach (see page 114)

1 Fry (sauté) the onion and carrots in the oil in a flameproof casserole (Dutch oven) for 2 minutes and remove with a draining spoon.

2 Add the chicken portions and fry quickly to brown on all sides. Drain off the excess fat.

3 Add the mushrooms, tomatoes, sherry, a little salt and pepper and the bouquet garni sachet.

4 Bring to the boil, cover and cook in a preheated oven at 180°C/350°F/gas mark 4 for 1½ hours. Remove the bouquet garni. Serve with Buttered Onion Spinach.

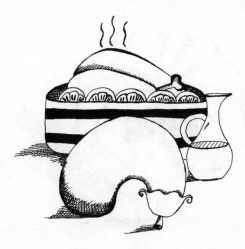

Chicken and Vegetable Stir-fry

SERVES 2

30 ml/2 tbsp sunflower oil
175 g/6 oz/1½ cups chicken stir-fry meat
¼ head Chinese leaves (stem lettuce), shredded
2 carrots, cut into matchsticks
100 g/4 oz mangetout (snow peas)
5 cm/2 in piece of cucumber, cut in matchsticks
1 bunch of spring onions (scallions), sliced
50 g/2 oz button mushrooms, sliced
½ red (bell) pepper, sliced
100 g/4 oz bean sprouts
5 ml/1 tsp grated fresh root ginger
½ garlic clove, crushed
Salt and freshly ground black pepper
30 ml/2 tbsp soy sauce
50 ml/2 fl oz/3½ tbsp water
¼ vegetable stock cube

1 Heat the oil in a wok or frying pan (skillet). Add the chicken and stir-fry for 3 minutes.

2 Add all the prepared vegetables except the bean sprouts and continue stir-frying for a further 5 minutes.

3 Add the bean sprouts and the other remaining ingredients and continue stir-frying for a further 3 minutes. Serve straight away.

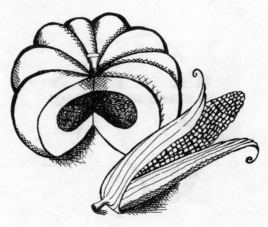

Marinated Tofu Salad

SERVES 4

250 g/9 oz packet firm tofu, drained and cubed
30 ml/2 tbsp soy sauce
45 ml/3 tbsp sherry
5 ml/1 tsp ground ginger
½ garlic clove, crushed
1.5 ml/¼ tsp chilli powder
30 ml/2 tbsp apple juice
100 g/4 oz button mushrooms, sliced
30 ml/2 tbsp olive oil
15 ml/1 tbsp lemon juice
Salt and freshly ground black pepper
½ iceberg lettuce, shredded
1.5 ml/¼ tsp dried thyme
2 carrots, coarsely grated
1 red (bell) pepper, diced
To garnish:
10 ml/2 tsp snipped chives

1 Put the tofu in a small, shallow dish.

2 Whisk together the next six ingredients and pour over. Toss well then cover and chill for 24 hours, if possible, tossing occasionally.

3 When ready to serve, put the button mushrooms in a salad bowl. Drizzle the oil and lemon juice over and add a little salt and pepper. Toss well.

4 Add the lettuce, thyme, carrots and pepper and toss again.

5 Lastly, add the tofu cubes and any remaining marinade, toss gently so as not to break them up, and sprinkle with chives.

Caesar Salad Special

SERVES 2

1 onion, sliced and separated into rings
30 ml/2 tbsp sunflower oil
2 eggs
45 ml/3 tbsp milk
Knob of butter
Freshly ground black pepper
4 anchovy fillets, drained
¼ iceberg lettuce, torn into pieces
12 stuffed olives, halved
15 ml/1 tbsp olive oil
10 ml/2 tsp lemon juice
2.5 ml/½ tsp mustard
To garnish:
Sliced tomatoes and cucumber

1 Fry (sauté) the onion rings in the sunflower oil until a rich golden brown. Remove from the pan with a draining spoon and drain on kitchen paper.

2 Beat the eggs with 30 ml/2 tbsp of the milk. Melt the butter in a small pan, add the eggs and a little pepper and cook, stirring until creamy but not too set. Remove from the heat and stand the base of the pan in cold water to prevent further cooking.

3 Soak the anchovy fillets in the remaining milk for 5 minutes then drain and chop.

4 Place the lettuce in a bowl. Add the eggs, anchovies and olives. Toss gently then pile into shallow bowls. Whisk the oil, lemon juice, mustard and a little pepper. Drizzle over the salad. Top with the onion rings and arrange slices of tomato and cucumber around.

Watercress Roulade

SERVES 2–3

1 onion, finely chopped
15 ml/1 tbsp olive oil
4 tomatoes, chopped
15 ml/1 tbsp tomato purée (paste)
1 bunch of watercress, chopped
15 ml/1 tbsp chopped parsley
45 ml/3 tbsp grated Parmesan cheese
Salt and freshly ground black pepper
4 eggs, separated
To serve:
Sesame Bean Sprout Salad (see page 118)

1 Fry (sauté) the onion in the oil for 2 minutes until soft but not brown. Add the tomatoes and tomato purée, cover and cook over a gentle heat for 5 minutes or until pulpy, stirring occasionally. Keep warm.

2 Mix the chopped watercress with the parsley and 30 ml/ 2 tbsp of the cheese. Season lightly.

3 Beat in the egg yolks. Whisk the egg whites until stiff and fold in with a metal spoon.

4 Spoon into a greased 18x28 cm/7x11 in Swiss roll tin (jelly roll pan), lined with greased greaseproof (waxed) paper. Level the surface.

5 Bake in a preheated oven at 200°C/400°F/gas mark 6 for about 10 minutes until golden and firm to the touch.

6 Dust another sheet of greaseproof paper with the remaining Parmesan. Carefully turn the roulade out on to the sheet and peel off the baking paper with the help of a knife.

7 Spread the warm tomato mixture over, then roll up using the greaseproof paper to help.

8 Transfer to a warm serving plate, cut in slices and serve with Sesame Bean Sprout Salad.

Fragrant Grilled Lamb with Tomatoes

SERVES 2

2 lamb leg steaks, trimmed of any fat
1 garlic clove, crushed
5 ml/1 tsp dried rosemary, crushed
25 g/1 oz/2 tbsp butter, softened
Salt and freshly ground black pepper
2 tomatoes, halved
To serve:
Braised Leeks (see page 114)

1 Lay the lamb steaks on a piece of foil on the grill (broiler) rack.

2 Mash the garlic with the rosemary and butter.

3 Spread half of the mixture over the lamb and season with salt and pepper.

4 Place under a hot grill for 4–5 minutes until golden brown and sizzling.

5 Turn over and spread with the remaining butter mixture. Add the tomatoes to the grill. Season the meat and the tomatoes.

6 Grill for a further 4–5 minutes until cooked through. Carefully transfer to warm serving plates, spooning the buttery juices over. Serve with Braised Leeks.

Lemon-glazed Lamb Cutlets

SERVES 2

4 lamb cutlets, trimmed of fat
Salt and freshly ground black pepper
20 g/¾ oz/1½ tbsp butter
Grated rind and juice of ½ lemon
45 ml/3 tbsp apple juice
To garnish:
Parsley sprigs
To serve:
Fruity Red Cabbage (see page 117)
Green beans

1 Season the cutlets with a little salt and pepper. Fry (sauté) in the butter in a frying pan (skillet) for 10 minutes until golden brown on each side and cooked through. Remove from the pan and keep warm.

2 Add the lemon rind, juice and the apple juice to the pan. Bring to the boil and boil rapidly until well reduced. Season to taste. Return the lamb to the pan and turn to coat in the juices.

3 Transfer to warm plates and garnish with parsley before serving with Fruity Red Cabbage and green beans.

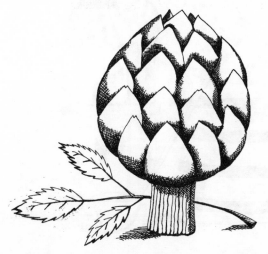

Beef Stroganoff

SERVES 2

1 onion, sliced
50 g/2 oz button mushrooms, sliced
25 g/1 oz/2 tbsp butter
225 g/8 oz fillet steak, cut in thin strips
Salt and freshly ground black pepper
15 ml/1 tbsp brandy (optional)
150 ml/¼ pt/⅔ cup soured (dairy sour) cream
30 ml/2 tbsp chopped parsley
To serve:
Broccoli and Cauliflower Stir-fry (see page 115)

1 Fry (sauté) the onion and mushrooms in the butter for 3 minutes, stirring.

2 Add the steak and continue to fry, stirring, for 4 minutes until the strips are just cooked.

3 Season well, stir in the brandy, if using, the soured cream and the parsley, and cook, stirring for 2–3 minutes until thickened. Taste and re-season if necessary. Serve straight away with Broccoli and Cauliflower Stir-fry.

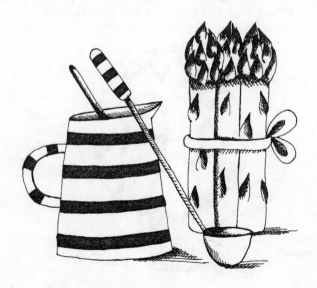

Grilled Sirloin Steak Sorrento

SERVES 2

2 sirloin steaks (about 175 g/6 oz each)
Salt and freshly ground black pepper
30 ml/2 tbsp olive oil
1 onion, sliced
1 red and 1 green (bell) pepper, sliced
1 aubergine (eggplant), sliced
6 black olives, halved
60 ml/4 tbsp red wine
1 tomato, skinned and finely chopped
Knob of butter
To serve:
Puréed Carrots and Peas (see page 116)

1 Trim any fat from the steaks. Place on a grill (broiler) rack and season. Brush with a little of the oil. Cook under a hot grill (broiler) for 3–4 minutes each side for medium and 5 minutes each side for well done – or according to preference.

2 Meanwhile, heat the remaining oil in a frying pan (skillet) and fry (sauté) the onion, peppers and aubergine for 8 minutes until tender. Add the olives and season to taste.

3 Put the steaks on warm plates, spoon the vegetable mixture on top and keep warm.

4 Add the wine and tomato to the pan and boil rapidly with the knob of butter, stirring for 2 minutes. Spoon over the steaks and serve with Puréed Carrots and Peas.

Braised Duck with Peas and Lettuce

SERVES 4

1 oven-ready duck (about 2 kg/4½ lb)
450 ml/¾ pt/2 cups stock made from the giblets or
   with vegetable stock cubes
30 ml/2 tbsp sunflower oil
Salt and freshly ground black pepper
225 g/8 oz shelled peas
30 ml/2 tbsp chopped mint
1.5 ml/¼ tsp grated nutmeg
1 round lettuce, shredded
To garnish:
Watercress sprigs
Orange segments
To serve:
Nutty Cauliflower (see page 116)

1 Remove the giblets from the duck and wipe the duck inside
and out with kitchen paper.

2 To make the stock, place the giblets in a pan with 600 ml/
1 pt/2½ cups water. Bring to the boil, reduce the heat, cover
and simmer for 30 minutes, then strain to make the stock.
Alternatively, make up the vegetable stock.

3 Meanwhile, prick the duck all over with a fork. Heat the oil
in a flameproof casserole (Dutch oven) and brown the duck
on all sides. Pour off all excess oil.

4 Add the measured amount of stock to the duck. Season
well. Cover, bring to the boil then cook in a preheated
oven at 180°C/350°F/gas mark 4 for 30 minutes.

5 Add the peas, mint, nutmeg and lettuce around the bird
and cook for a further 1½ hours until the duck is really
tender.

6 Remove the duck and cut in quarters. Spoon off any fat
from the juices then boil rapidly until reduced by half.
Taste and re-season if necessary. Spoon over the duck.

7 Garnish with the watercress and orange segments and
serve with Nutty Cauliflower.

Normandy Pheasant

SERVES 2

1 large onion, sliced
40 g/1½ oz/3 tbsp butter
1 oven-ready hen pheasant
Salt and freshly ground black pepper
150 ml/¼ pt/⅔ cup cider
150 ml/¼ pt/⅔ cup double (heavy) cream
1 eating (dessert) apple
Lemon juice
To garnish:
Snipped chives
To serve:
Mixed Green Salad (see page 123)

1 Fry (sauté) the onion in the butter in a flameproof casserole for 2 minutes, stirring. Add the pheasant and brown on all sides.

2 Season all over and add the cider. Bring to the boil, cover and cook in a preheated oven at 180°C/350°F/gas mark 4 for 1 hour.

3 Remove the pheasant and split in half. Keep warm.

4 Add the cream to the juices in the pan, bring to the boil and cook, stirring, until thickened. Season to taste.

5 Core and thinly slice the apple but do not peel. Dip in lemon juice to prevent browning. Spoon the sauce over the pheasant and arrange the apple slices attractively to one side.

6 Garnish with snipped chives and serve straight away with Mixed Green Salad.

CARBOHYDRATE-RICH

Carbohydrate-rich meals tend to be more filling than protein-rich ones and 'bulkier'. You may find you don't need to fill up with quite so much salad and vegetables as with the protein meals. On the whole, they digest well and can be eaten at whatever time of day suits you best – though I don't advocate eating late at night and then going straight to bed!

Country Vegetable Broth

SERVES 4

1 onion, coarsely grated
3 carrots, coarsely grated
1 parsnip, coarsely grated
4 celery sticks, grated
1 turnip, coarsely grated
1 potato, coarsely grated
40 g/1½ oz/3 tbsp butter
1.5 litres/2½ pts/6 cups vegetable stock
Salt and freshly ground black pepper
100 g/4 oz/good ½ cup pearl barley
1 bouquet garni sachet
To garnish:
30 ml/2 tbsp chopped parsley
To serve:
Wholemeal rolls (optional)

1 Fry (sauté) all the prepared vegetables in the butter in a large saucepan for 3 minutes, stirring.

2 Add the stock, some salt and pepper, the barley and bouquet garni sachet. Bring to the boil, part cover, reduce the heat and simmer gently for 1 hour or until the barley is tender.

3 Discard the bouquet garni sachet. Ladle into soup bowls and sprinkle with chopped parsley before serving with a wholemeal roll each, if liked.

Spiced Bulgar with Pine Nuts

SERVES 2

1 onion, finely chopped,
1 small garlic clove, crushed
10 ml/2 tsp olive oil
50 g/2 oz/½ cup bulgar wheat
1.5 ml/¼ tsp ground coriander (cilantro)
Good pinch of ground cinnamon
Pinch of chilli powder
300 ml/½ pt/1¼ cups vegetable stock
Salt and freshly ground black pepper
50 g/2 oz/⅓ cup raisins
75 g/3 oz/¾ cup pine nuts
Salt and freshly ground black pepper
15 ml/1 tbsp chopped parsley
2 tomatoes, chopped
5 cm/2 in piece of cucumber, chopped
5 ml/1 tsp dried mint

1 Fry (sauté) the onion and garlic in the oil in a saucepan for 2 minutes, stirring.

2 Stir in the remaining ingredients except the parsley, tomatoes, cucumber and mint, seasoning lightly.

3 Cover, reduce the heat and cook gently for 20 minutes until the liquid is absorbed and the wheat is soft. Fluff up with a fork and stir in the parsley. Taste and add more seasoning if necessary. Mix the tomato and cucumber together with the mint.

4 Pile on to plates and top with the tomato and cucumber mixture. Serve straight away.

Spinach and Cashew Nut Parcels

SERVES 2

225 g/8 oz spinach
1 onion, roughly chopped
15 g/½ oz/1 tbsp butter
75 g/3 oz/¾ cup cashew nuts
2 slices wholemeal bread
1 egg yolk
150 ml/¼ pt/⅔ cup hot water
5 ml/1 tsp yeast extract
1.5 ml/¼ tsp dried oregano
Salt and freshly ground black pepper
½ vegetable stock cube
5 ml/1 tsp cornflour (cornstarch)
To serve:
Jacket potatoes
Tomato, Chive and Carrot Salad (see page 124)

1 Wash the spinach very well, reserve six of the largest leaves and tear the remainder into pieces, discarding thick stalks.

2 Cook the torn spinach in a saucepan without any extra water for 5 minutes in a covered pan. Drain off any liquid.

3 Fry (sauté) the onion in the butter for 3 minutes, stirring. Put in a food processor with the cooked spinach, the nuts and the bread. Run the machine briefly until finely chopped but not puréed.

4 Mix the egg yolk with 30 ml/2 tbsp of the water and the yeast extract. Add to the processor with the oregano and some salt and pepper and run the machine very briefly to bind the mixture together.

5 Trim any thick stalks from the remaining six spinach leaves. Plunge in boiling water for 20 seconds and drain. Lay on a board.

6 Divide the nut mixture between the spinach leaves, fold over the edges and roll up to form parcels. Pack in the base of a flameproof casserole (Dutch oven). Blend the remaining water with the stock cube and pour around.

7 Cook in a preheated oven at 180°C/350°F/gas mark 4 for 35 minutes.

8 Carefully remove from the casserole with a draining spoon and place on serving plates. Blend the cornflour with 15 ml/1 tbsp water and stir into the stock in the pan. Bring to the boil and cook for 1 minute, stirring. Spoon over the parcels and serve with jacket potatoes and Tomato, Chive and Carrot Salad.

Vegetable Risotto

SERVES 2

1 onion, chopped
100 g/4 oz broccoli, cut in tiny florets
½ small cauliflower, cut in small florets
1 carrot, diced
1 small red (bell) pepper, diced
75 g/3 oz shelled peas
75 g/3 oz sweetcorn (corn)
25 g/1 oz/2 tbsp butter
100 g/4 oz/½ cup brown rice
600 ml/1 pt/2½ cups vegetable stock
Salt and freshly ground black pepper
1 bouquet garni sachet
15 ml/1 tbsp chopped parsley
15 ml/1 tbsp snipped chives

1 Fry (sauté) the vegetables in the butter, stirring for 2 minutes.

2 Stir in the rice and cook for 1 minute. Add the stock, some salt and pepper and the bouquet garni and bring to the boil.

3 Cover and cook in a preheated oven at 200°C/400°F/gas mark 6 for 35–40 minutes or until the rice has absorbed the liquid and the vegetables are tender.

4 Stir in the parsley and chives and serve.

Root Vegetable Pasties with Creamed Mushroom Sauce

MAKES 4

350 g/12 oz/3 cups wholemeal flour,
  plus extra for dusting
Pinch of salt
200 g/ 7 oz/scant 1 cup butter
15 ml/1 tbsp fennel seeds
Cold water to mix
1 potato, finely diced
2 carrots, finely diced
½ small swede (rutabaga), finely diced
1 small parsnip, finely diced
1 onion, finely chopped
Freshly ground black pepper
7.5 ml/1½ tsp yeast extract
30 ml/2 tbsp hot water
325 ml/11 fl oz/1⅓ cups single (light) cream
75 g/3 oz button mushrooms, sliced
15 ml/1 tbsp cornflour (cornstarch)
2.5 ml/½ tsp dried mixed herbs
To serve:
Mixed Leaf Salad (see page 126)

1 Mix the flour and salt in a bowl.

2 Add 175 g/6 oz/¾ cup of the butter, cut into small pieces, and rub in with the fingertips until the mixture resembles breadcrumbs.

3 Stir in the fennel seeds then mix with enough cold water to form a firm dough.

4 Knead gently on a lightly floured surface. Roll out to a rectangle and cut into quarters.

5 Mix the prepared vegetables together in a bowl, seasoning well. Spoon on to the centres of the pastry squares. Blend the yeast extract with the water and spoon over each pile of vegetables. Brush the edges of the pastry with a little water and fold over the filling to form oblong parcels. Knock up the edges and flute with the back of a knife. Make a tiny slit in the top of each with the point of a knife to allow steam to escape.

6 Transfer to a baking sheet and brush with a little of the single cream to glaze. Bake in a preheated oven at 190°C/375°F/gas mark 5 for about 45 minutes until well browned and the vegetables are tender.

7 Meanwhile make the sauce. Melt the remaining butter in a saucepan. Add the mushrooms and fry (sauté) stirring for 3 minutes. Remove from the heat and stir in the cornflour. Blend in the remaining cream and the herbs. Bring to the boil and cook for 1 minute, stirring. Season to taste. Serve the pasties warm with the sauce and Mixed Leaf Salad.

Rotelli with Broccoli and Cream

SERVES 2

100 g/4 oz wholemeal rotelli
  (or other pasta shapes)
175 g/6 oz broccoli, cut in tiny florets
1 onion, finely chopped
1 garlic clove, crushed
15 g/½ oz/1 tbsp butter
15 ml/1 tbsp olive oil
150 ml/¼ pt/⅔ cup single (light) cream
Salt and freshly ground black pepper
To garnish:
Cayenne
To serve:
Peasant Mixed Salad (see page 119)

1 Cook the pasta in boiling, lightly salted water according to the packet directions. Add the broccoli for the last 5 minutes of cooking time. Drain and return to the saucepan.

2 Meanwhile, fry (sauté) the onion, and garlic in the butter and oil for 3 minutes until softened but not browned.

3 Add to the pasta with the cream and toss well over a gentle heat. Pile on to plates and sprinkle with cayenne before serving with Peasant Mixed Salad.

Tagliatelle with Corn and Mushrooms

SERVES 2

100 g/4 oz wholemeal tagliatelle
100 g/4 oz baby corn cobs
15 g/½ oz/1 tbsp butter
1 small onion, chopped
1 small garlic clove, crushed
75 g /3 oz button mushrooms, sliced
90 ml/6 tbsp single (light) cream
Salt and freshly ground black pepper
5 ml/1 tsp chopped thyme
10 ml/2 tsp chopped parsley
To serve:
Wholemeal bread (optional)
Green salad

1 Cook the tagliatelle according to the packet directions, adding the corn for the last 4 minutes of cooking time. Drain and return to the pan.

2 Meanwhile, melt the butter in a separate pan and fry (sauté) the onion, garlic and mushrooms for 5 minutes, stirring until soft but not brown.

3 Add to the pasta and corn with the cream, some salt and pepper and the herbs. Toss gently, pile on to plates and serve with wholemeal bread, if liked, and a green salad.

Pasta with Green Beans and Basil

SERVES 2

175 g/6 oz wholemeal spaghetti
100 g/4 oz French beans, cut in short lengths
Handful of basil leaves, chopped
1 small garlic clove
25 g/1 oz/2 tbsp butter
15 ml/1 tbsp olive oil
45 ml/3 tbsp pine nuts
Salt and freshly ground black pepper

1 Cook the pasta according to the packet directions, and add the beans for the last 5 minutes of cooking time. Drain and return to the saucepan.

2 Meanwhile, blend the basil, garlic, butter, oil and pine nuts with a little salt and plenty of pepper in a blender or food processor, stopping the machine and scraping down the sides as necessary.

3 Add to the cooked pasta and beans and toss over a gentle heat until piping hot. Serve straight away.

Savoury Spinach Layer

SERVES 2

350 g/12 oz spinach, torn in pieces
1 onion, sliced
20 ml/4 tsp oil
4 slices wholemeal bread, crusts removed
Home-made Sesame Butter (see page 156)
Salt and freshly ground black pepper
Grated nutmeg
To serve:
Lightly cooked carrots

1 Wash the spinach well, shake off excess water then cook in a covered saucepan with no extra water for 5 minutes. Drain and chop.

2 Fry (sauté) the onion in half the oil until soft. Remove from the pan with a draining spoon and mix with the spinach.

3 Make one of the slices of bread into breadcrumbs and put to one side. Spread the remaining slices with Sesame Butter. Put 1½ slices in the base of an oiled, shallow ovenproof dish, nutty side up.

4 Season the spinach mixture with salt, pepper and nutmeg. Spread half over the bread. Top with the remaining bread slices and then the remaining spinach mixture.

5 Melt 15 ml/1 tbsp peanut butter with the remaining oil and stir in the breadcrumbs. Scatter over the spinach and bake in a preheated oven at 190°C/375°F/gas mark 5 until piping hot and the top is golden brown. Serve with lightly cooked carrots.

Vegetable Fajitas

SERVES 2

Chilli Salsa:
4 ripe tomatoes, skinned and chopped
1 small onion, finely chopped
2 fresh green chillies, seeded and finely chopped
1 small garlic clove, crushed
45 ml/3 tbsp chopped coriander (cilantro) leaves
Salt and freshly ground black pepper
Cornmeal Pancakes:
100 g/4 oz/1 cup wholemeal flour
1.5 ml/¼ tsp salt
50 g/2 oz/½ cup cornmeal
400 ml/14 fl oz/1¾ cups water
1 egg yolk
A little sunflower oil for greasing
Filling:
60 ml/4 tbsp olive oil
1 small aubergine (eggplant), sliced
1 red (bell) pepper, cut into strips
1 red onion, sliced
1 courgette (zucchini), sliced
100 g/4 oz button mushrooms, quartered

1 Make the chilli salsa first by mixing together all the ingredients, adding seasoning to taste.

2 Beat the pancake ingredients together in a bowl until smooth, adding a little extra water if necessary, to form a thick pouring batter.

3 Heat a little oil in a small frying pan (skillet). Pour off the excess then add about 45 ml/3 tbsp of the batter and swirl round to coat the base thickly. Cook over a moderate heat until the pancake is dry but the edges are not brown. Turn over and cook the other side briefly. Slide out of the pan on to a plate over a pan of hot water and cook the remaining pancakes in the same way.

4 Make the filling. Heat the oil in a large frying pan and fry (sauté) the prepared vegetables, stirring for 6–8 minutes until soft and lightly golden. Season with salt and pepper.

5 Divide the vegetable mixture between the pancakes. Top with a little chilli salsa, roll up and eat.

Mexican Rice

SERVES 2

15 g/½ oz/1 tbsp butter
1 garlic clove, crushed
1 small red (bell) pepper, diced
1 small green (bell) pepper, diced
½ bunch of spring onions (scallions), chopped
1 carrot, diced
100 g/4 oz/½ cup brown rice
2.5 ml/½ tsp chilli powder
375 g/13 fl oz/1½ cups vegetable stock
Salt and freshly ground black pepper
2 bananas, cut into chunks
15 ml/1 tbsp sunflower oil
8 stuffed olives, halved
To garnish:
Chopped parsley

1 Melt the butter in a large frying pan (skillet). Fry (sauté) the garlic, peppers, spring onions and carrot for 2 minutes, stirring.

2 Add the rice and chilli powder and cook for 1 minute, stirring.

3 Add the stock and a little salt and pepper. Bring to the boil, cover, reduce the heat and cook very gently for 35 minutes or until the rice has absorbed the liquid and is just tender but still nutty. Add a little water if necessary.

4 When nearly cooked fry the banana chunks in the oil in a separate pan. Stir the olives into the rice.

5 Spoon on to two plates, top with the banana then garnish with parsley before serving.

Stuffed Cabbage with Creamed Potatoes

SERVES 2

4 good-sized Savoy cabbage leaves (use the dark
  green outer ones)
100g/4 oz mushrooms
1 small onion, quartered
1 carrot, grated
100 g/4 oz /½ cup Mascarpone cheese
50 g/2 oz/1 cup wholemeal breadcrumbs
100 g/4 oz/1 cup chopped mixed nuts
Pinch of ground cinnamon
Salt and freshly ground black pepper
300 ml/½ pt/1¼ cups boiling water
1 vegetable stock cube
450 g/1 lb potatoes, scrubbed
Knob of butter
30 ml/2 tbsp single (light) cream
10 ml/2 tsp cornflour (cornstarch)
To garnish:
Chopped parsley

1 Cut out any thick central core from the cabbage leaves.
Plunge in boiling water for 1 minute then drain, rinse with
cold water and drain again. Dry on kitchen paper.

2 Put the mushrooms, onion, carrot, cheese, breadcrumbs,
nuts, cinnamon and some salt and pepper in a blender or food
processor and run the machine until the mixture forms a ball.

3 Divide between the cabbage leaves, fold in the sides and roll
up to form parcels. Pack into a small flameproof casserole
(Dutch oven).

4 Mix the water and stock cube together. Pour around. Bring to
the boil, cover, reduce the heat and cook for 15–20 minutes
or until the cabbage is tender.

5 Meanwhile cook the potatoes in boiling, lightly salted water
until tender. Drain and remove the skins.

6 Mash the potatoes with the butter and cream until fluffy and
season to taste.

7 Carefully lift the cooked stuffed cabbage out on to warm plates and keep warm. Blend the cornflour with a little cold water and stir into the juices in the pan. Bring to the boil and cook for 1 minute until thickened.

8 Pour over the cabbage and serve with the creamed potatoes, garnished with parsley.

Hot Potato Sauté

SERVES 2

450 g/1 lb new potatoes, scrubbed and cut into bite-sized pieces
50 g/2 oz/¼ cup butter
1 bunch of spring onions (scallions), chopped
1 each small green and red (bell) pepper, chopped
175 g/6 oz sweetcorn (corn)
5 cm/2 in piece cucumber, diced
Salt and freshly ground black pepper
2.5 ml/½ tsp dried oregano
To serve:
Green Bean and Tomato Salad (see page 124)

1 Cook the potatoes in boiling, lightly salted water for about 8 minutes or until tender. Drain.

2 Melt the butter in a wok or large frying pan (skillet). Add the spring onions, peppers and the potatoes and fry (sauté), stirring for 5 minutes or until the vegetables are turning golden.

3 Add the remaining ingredients and continue cooking for 3 minutes, stirring until piping hot and the cucumber is cooked but still has some 'bite'. Serve straight away with Green Bean and Tomato Salad.

Mexican Avocado Salad

SERVES 2

100 g/4 oz wholemeal macaroni
1 vegetable stock cube
5 ml/1 tsp powdered saffron
100 g/4 oz frozen sweetcorn (corn)
1 red onion, chopped
1 green (bell) pepper, chopped
2 tomatoes, roughly cut up
1 avocado, peeled and diced
Crisp lettuce leaves
Dressing:
2 ripe tomatoes, skinned and chopped
30 ml/2 tbsp olive oil
Salt and freshly ground black pepper
15 ml/1 tbsp chopped parsley
1 green chilli, chopped
1 small garlic clove, chopped

1 Cook the macaroni according to packet directions, adding the stock cube and saffron to the boiling water. Add the sweetcorn for the last 5 minutes of cooking time. Drain and leave to cool.

2 Place in a bowl with the onion, pepper, tomatoes and avocado. Season and mix gently. Pile into shallow bowls, lined with crisp lettuce leaves.

3 Blend the dressing ingredients together in a blender or food processor until smooth. Drizzle over and serve.

NEUTRAL

All of these are ideal to eat at lunch time or in the evening. They can be turned into protein meals by adding some fish, cheese or meat or into carbohydrate meals by eating with wholemeal bread, or adding some potatoes, rice or pasta.

Curried Vegetables with Coconut

SERVES 2

10 ml/2 tsp sunflower oil
1 bay leaf
Small piece of cinnamon stick
5 cardamom pods, split
3 cloves
10 ml/2 tsp ground coriander (cilantro)
10 ml/2 tsp ground cumin
Pinch of chilli powder
5 ml/1 tsp turmeric
1 garlic clove, crushed
1 small onion, chopped
2 carrots, diced
1 parsnip, diced
50 g/2 oz green beans, cut into short lengths
1 courgette (zucchini), diced
50 g/2 oz shelled peas
150 ml/¼ pt/⅔ cup vegetable stock
50 g/2 oz/½ cup creamed coconut
7.5 ml/1½ tsp garam masala
Salt and freshly ground black pepper
To serve:
A few torn coriander (cilantro) leaves

1 Heat the oil in a saucepan and fry (sauté) the bay leaf and spices for 1 minute. Add the garlic and onion and fry for 2 minutes. Add the vegetables and stock.

2 Bring to the boil, reduce the heat, part-cover and simmer gently for about 30 minutes or until the vegetables are really tender and the liquid is reduced by half.

3 Stir in the coconut and garam masala. Taste and reseason.

4 Sprinkle with coriander leaves and serve (take care not to eat the pieces of spices!).

Mediterranean-style Grilled Mixed Peppers

SERVES 2

**1 each of red, yellow, green and orange (bell)
    peppers, cut into quarters**
90 ml/6 tbsp olive oil
2 garlic cloves, crushed
Pinch of cayenne
15 ml/1 tbsp chopped fresh basil
Coarse sea salt
12 black olives
To serve:
Mixed Green Salad (see page 123)

1 Lay the peppers on a sheet of foil on the grill (broiler) rack.

2 Whisk the oil with the garlic, cayenne and basil. Brush over the peppers.

3 Grill (broil) for about 10 minutes until tender, turning frequently and brushing with more flavoured oil.

4 Place on warm serving plates, drizzle any remaining oil over and sprinkle with coarse sea salt and the olives. Serve with Mixed Green Salad.

Tangy Chestnut Kebabs

SERVES 2

**225 g/8 oz fresh cooked or canned chestnuts,
    drained**
60 ml/4 tbsp butter, melted
15 ml/1 tbsp grated orange rind
5 ml/1 tsp grated lemon rind

1 Thread the chestnuts on to skewers. Place on foil on the grill (broiler) rack.

2 Mix the butter with the fruit rinds. Brush over the kebabs and grill (broil) for 5 minutes, turning frequently and brushing with more flavoured butter. Serve with any remaining flavoured butter drizzled over.

Root Vegetable Satay

SERVES 2

1 turnip, cut into bite-sized chunks
2 carrots, cut into bite-sized chunks
1 parsnip, cut into bite-sized chunks
¼ small swede (rutabaga), cut into bite-sized
   chunks
30 ml/2 tbsp melted butter
1 garlic clove, crushed
Peanut sauce:
100 ml/3½ fl oz/6½ tbsp single (light) cream
60 ml/4 tbsp Home-made Sesame Butter
   (see page 156)
1.5 ml/¼ tsp chilli powder (or less to taste)
30 ml/2 tbsp toasted sesame seeds

1 Cook the vegetables together in boiling, salted water until just tender (about 6 minutes). Drain, rinse with cold water and drain again.

2 Thread alternately on skewers.

3 Lay on foil on a grill (broiler) rack. Mix the butter and garlic together and brush all over the kebabs. Grill (broil) until golden, brushing frequently with the garlic butter.

4 Meanwhile, heat the cream and sesame butter together in a small pan with the chilli powder, stirring until smooth. Thin with a little water, if necessary. Spoon into two individual small bowls. Sprinkle with toasted sesame seeds and serve with the kebabs.

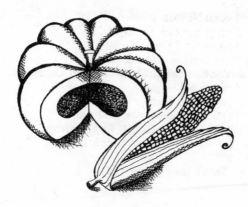

Gingered Vegetable Stir-fry

SERVES 2

1 aubergine (eggplant), diced
2 courgettes (zucchini), sliced
1 bunch of spring onions (scallions), sliced
    diagonally
1 yellow (bell) pepper, diced
2 carrots, sliced diagonally
50 g/2 oz mushrooms, sliced
2 garlic cloves, crushed
1.5 ml/¼ tsp ground cloves
1.5 ml/¼ tsp dried basil
5 ml/1 tsp grated fresh root ginger
1 stalk of lemon grass, very finely chopped
60 ml/4 tbsp olive oil
Salt and freshly ground black pepper
5 ml/1 tsp yeast extract
75 ml/5 tbsp boiling water
To garnish:
Tomato wedges

1 Stir-fry all the prepared vegetables in the oil with the garlic, cloves, basil, ginger and lemon grass in a wok or large frying pan (skillet) for 8 minutes.

2 Season well. Blend the yeast extract with the boiling water and add. Boil rapidly for 2 minutes until reduced by half. Serve piping hot, garnished with wedges of tomato.

Mushroom and Courgette Kebabs

SERVES 2

225 g/8 oz button mushrooms
3–4 courgettes (zucchini) cut into chunks
A little olive oil
50 g/2 oz/¼ cup butter
15 ml/1 tbsp toasted sesame seeds
1 spring onion (scallion), finely chopped
Salt and freshly ground black pepper
To serve:
Athena Salad (see page 122)

1 Thread the mushrooms and courgettes alternately on skewers.

2 Brush with a little oil and grill (broil) for about 10 minutes under a moderate grill (broiler), turning and brushing with oil frequently.

3 Melt the butter and stir in the sesame seeds, spring onion and a little salt and pepper.

4 Slide the kebabs on to serving plates and drizzle the sesame butter over. Serve with Athena Salad.

Vegetable Dolmas

SERVES 2

2 carrots, diced
100 g/4 oz broad (lima) beans
100 g/4 oz shelled peas
1 turnip, diced
Salt and freshly ground black pepper
Pinch of ground cinnamon
2.5 ml/½ tsp dried oregano
8 vine leaves from a packet, rinsed and dried
5 ml/1 tsp yeast extract
150 ml/¼ pt/⅔ cup water
150 ml/¼ pt/⅔ cup soured (dairy sour) cream
To garnish:
Chopped parsley
6 black olives

1 Cook the vegetables together in boiling, salted water until tender. Drain and mash slightly. Season with pepper, the cinnamon and the oregano.

2 Lay the vine leaves on a board. Divide the vegetable mixture between the leaves. Fold in the sides and roll up. Pack in a single layer in a flameproof casserole (Dutch oven).

3 Blend the yeast extract with the water and pour over. Bring to the boil, cover and bake in a preheated oven at 180°C/350°F/gas mark 4 for 30 minutes.

4 Transfer the dolmas to warm plates. Blend the soured cream into the juices and bubble for 2 minutes to thicken. Spoon over and garnish with parsley and olives.

Spiced Vegetable Casserole

SERVES 2

20 ml/4 tsp sunflower oil
1 onion, chopped
1 garlic clove, crushed
15 ml/1 tbsp curry powder
1 small red (bell) pepper, cut in chunks
1 green chilli, seeded and sliced
1 celery stick, cut in chunks
50 g/2 oz green beans, cut in pieces
50 g/2 oz shelled peas
1 carrot, diced
1 turnip, diced
1 bunch of spring onions (scallions), cut in
    diagonal slices
100 g/4 oz broad (lima) beans
100 g/4 oz broccoli, cut into small florets
600 ml/1 pt/2½ cups vegetable stock
1 bouquet garni sachet
Salt and freshly ground black pepper
To garnish:
Chopped parsley

1 Heat the oil in a large flameproof casserole (Dutch oven) and fry (sauté) the onion, garlic and curry powder for 2 minutes, stirring.

2 Add the remaining ingredients. Bring to the boil, cover and cook over a moderate heat for 20–30 minutes until the vegetables are tender. Remove the lid after 15 minutes to allow a little of the liquid to evaporate. Discard the bouquet garni sachet.

3 Serve in large soup bowls, sprinkled with chopped parsley.

Vegetable Terrine

SERVES 4

225 g/8 oz baby carrots, trimmed but left whole
100g/4 oz thin asparagus tips, tied in a bundle
225 g/8 oz French beans, cut in halves
100 g/4 oz broad (lima) beans
4 tomatoes, skinned, quartered and seeded
1½ sachets powdered gelatine or vegetarian
**   equivalent**
900 ml/1½ pts/3¾ cups vegetable stock
15 ml/1 tbsp chopped parsley
10 ml/2 tsp chopped thyme
A little oil
To serve:
Green salad

1 Cook the vegetables separately in boiling salted water until just
tender – take care not to overcook (especially the asparagus or
the heads will fall off). Drain, rinse with cold water and drain
again.

2 Soften the gelatine in a little of the stock, then heat until almost
boiling, stirring until clear. Do not allow to boil (or follow
directions for a vegetarian equivalent). Stir in the remaining
stock and the herbs.

3 Oil a 900 g/2 lb loaf tin (pan) and spoon about 5 mm/¼ in of the
stock mixture into the base. Chill until set.

4 Layer the vegetables attractively in the tin remembering that the
pattern on the base will show up when the terrine is turned out.

5 When the remaining jellied stock is almost the consistency of
egg white, carefully pour into the tin to cover the vegetables
completely. Chill until firm.

6 Carefully loosen the edges then turn out on to a serving dish
and serve with a green salad.

Avocado Salad with Rosy Dressing

SERVES 2

2 small avocados, halved, peeled and
  stoned (pitted)
Crisp lettuce leaves
5 cm/2 in piece of cucumber, grated
1 carrot, grated
10 ml/2 tsp poppy seeds
Dressing:
1 cooked beetroot (red beet)
¼ small onion
150 ml/¼ pt/⅔ cup soured (dairy sour) cream
Salt and freshly ground black pepper
To garnish:
Snipped chives

1 Lay the avocado halves cut sides down on a bed of lettuce on two serving plates.

2 Mix the cucumber, carrot and poppy seeds together and spoon around the edges.

3 To make the dressing, purée the beetroot and onion in a blender or food processor until smooth. Blend in the soured cream and season to taste.

4 Spoon over the avocados and sprinkle with snipped chives before serving.

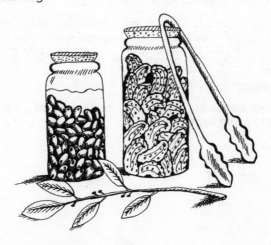

Turkish Aubergine Slippers

SERVES 2

1 large aubergine (eggplant)
Salt and freshly ground black pepper
45 ml/3 tbsp olive oil
1 large onion, chopped
1 garlic clove, crushed
Good pinch of ground cinnamon
15 ml/1 tbsp chopped parsley
15 ml/1 tbsp pine nuts, chopped
3 large tomatoes, skinned and finely chopped
To serve:
Mixed Leaf Salad (see page 126)

1 Cut the stalk off the aubergine and cook in boiling, salted water for 10 minutes. Drain and cover with cold water for 5 minutes to cool.

2 Cut in half and scoop out most of the flesh, leaving a thickish shell. Place the shells in an oiled ovenproof dish and season with a little salt and pepper. Drizzle with 15 ml/1 tbsp of the oil, cover with foil and bake in a preheated oven at 180°C/350°F/gas mark 4 for 30 minutes. Remove from the oven and leave until cold.

3 Meanwhile, chop the aubergine flesh. Heat the remaining oil in a frying pan (skillet) and fry (sauté) the onion and garlic for 5 minutes until soft and lightly golden. Stir in the cinnamon, parsley, chopped aubergine flesh and pine nuts. Cook gently for 15 minutes or until pulpy, stirring occasionally. Season to taste and leave to cool.

4 When cold, stir in the chopped tomato and pile into the shells. Serve with Mixed Leaf Salad.

Spinach Mousse

SERVES 4

450 g/1 lb spinach
50 g/2 oz/¼ cup butter
1 onion, chopped
8 basil leaves
15 ml/1 tbsp powdered gelatine
5 ml/1 tsp grated nutmeg
Salt and freshly ground black pepper
300 ml/½ pt/1¼ cups double (heavy) cream
To serve:
Rainbow Salad (see page 119)

1 Discard any tough stalks from the spinach. Wash thoroughly, shake off excess moisture.

2 Melt the butter in a saucepan. Add the onion and cook gently for 2 minutes until soft but not brown.

3 Add the spinach, stir until it starts to cook down, then cover and cook gently for 10 minutes.

4 Throw in the basil leaves. Tilt the pan so the juices run to one side. Sprinkle the gelatine into these and stir until dissolved. Purée in a blender or food processor.

5 Stir in the nutmeg and some salt and pepper.

6 Whip the cream until peaking. Fold into the purée with a metal spoon. Turn into an oiled mould (mold) or attractive glass dish. Chill until set. Turn out, if necessary, and serve with Rainbow Salad.

Mushroom Pâté-stuffed Peppers

SERVES 2

4 small (bell) peppers, any colour
1 small onion, finely chopped
25 g/1 oz/2 tbsp butter
350 g/12 oz mushrooms, finely chopped
225 g/8 oz/1 cup Mascarpone cheese
30 ml/2 tbsp chopped parsley
Salt and freshly ground black pepper
To serve:
Village Garden Salad (see page 120)

1 Cut a slice off the tops of the peppers and discard the seeds. Trim the bases so they stand up, taking care not to make holes. Plunge the peppers and lids in boiling water for 1 minute. Drain, rinse with cold water, drain again and dry with kitchen paper.

2 Fry (sauté) the onion in the butter for 3 minutes until a pale golden brown.

3 Add the mushrooms and fry until no liquid remains, stirring all the time.

4 Turn into a bowl and leave until cold.

5 Beat in the cheese and parsley and season to taste.

6 Spoon into the peppers, top with the lids and chill until firm. Serve cold with Village Garden Salad.

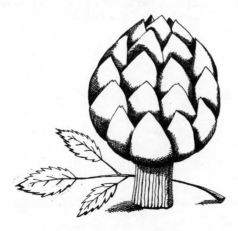

Russian Salad Deluxe

SERVES 2

2 carrots, diced
1 parsnip, diced
1 turnip, diced
75 g/3 oz shelled peas
Mayonnaise:
1 egg yolk
Salt and freshly ground black pepper
Grated rind of 1 lemon
150 ml/¼ pt/⅔ cup olive oil
To garnish:
4 cooked beetroot (red beets), sliced
Snipped chives

1 Cook the carrots, parsnip and turnip in boiling, salted water for about 8–10 minutes until tender. Add the peas after 5 minutes. Drain, rinse with cold water and drain again.

2 Make the mayonnaise. Put the egg yolk in a bowl with a little salt and pepper and the lemon rind. Whisk to mix. Then gradually add the oil a drop at a time, whisking well until thick and glossy. Taste and add more seasoning if necessary.

3 Add half the mayonnnaise to the vegetables and fold in. (Store the remainder in a screw-topped jar in the fridge for up to one week.)

4 Pile on to two plates. Arrange the beetroot slices all round the edge and sprinkle with snipped chives before serving.

Summer Salad Platter

SERVES 2

100 g/4 oz thin asparagus spears, tied in a bundle
1 head of chicory (Belgian endive)
1 bunch of radishes, trimmed
8 cherry tomatoes
5 cm/2 in piece cucumber, diced
100 g/4 oz fresh shelled peas
1 small leek, thinly sliced
Dressing:
3 ripe tomatoes, skinned, seeded (pitted)
  and chopped
30 ml/2 tbsp olive or sunflower oil
Salt and freshly ground black pepper
30 ml/2 tbsp single (light) cream
Grated rind of ½ lemon

1 Stand the asparagus in a pan with enough boiling water to come half-way up the stems. Cover and cook for 5 minutes then turn off the heat and leave to stand until cold.

2 Cut a cone-shaped central core out of the chicory then separate into leaves.

3 Arrange all the vegetables attractively on a platter.

4 Blend the dressing ingredients together in a blender or food processor until smooth. Pour into a small jug and serve with the salad.

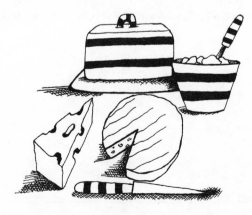

Shredded Vegetable Platter with Soured Cream Dressing

SERVES 2

If you don't have a vegetable shredder, use the coarse blade of a grater.

2 carrots, thinly shredded
1 head of celeriac (celery root) thinly shredded
2 turnips, thinly shredded
2 courgettes (zucchini), thinly shredded
2 beetroot (red beets), thinly shredded
6 black olives, chopped
Dressing:
150 ml/¼ pt/⅔ cup soured (dairy sour) cream
15 ml/1 tbsp olive oil
5 ml/1 tsp curry powder
Salt and freshly ground black pepper
A little water
To garnish:
30 ml/2 tbsp sunflower seeds

1 Arrange the different vegetables in piles attractively on two serving plates.

2 Whisk the dressing ingredients together, thinning with a little water if necessary.

3 Drizzle over and sprinkle with sunflower seeds. Serve straight away.

Salads and Vegetables

The following recipes are almost all neutral and can be served with absolutely any meal you like. The exception is Fruity Red Cabbage which must be served as part of a protein-rich meal. When you are serving any of the snacks as part of a protein meal you may spike the dressing with lemon juice if you like.

Minted Peas and Lettuce

SERVES 2

100 g/4 oz fresh, shelled peas
½ small hearty lettuce, cut in 4 wedges
60 ml/4 tbsp boiling water
¼ vegetable stock cube
25 g/1 oz/2 tbsp butter, softened
15 ml/1 tbsp chopped mint

1 Put the peas and lettuce in a small flameproof casserole (Dutch oven). Mix the water with the stock cube and add to the vegetables. Cover and cook over a gentle heat for 10 minutes. Remove the lid after 5 minutes.

2 Mash the butter with the mint and add to the pan. Cover and cook for 1 minute more. Serve straight away.

Buttered Onion Spinach

SERVES 2

2 onions, sliced into rings
25 g/1 oz/2 tbsp butter
350 g/12 oz spinach
45 ml/3 tbsp double (heavy) cream
2.5 ml/½ tsp grated nutmeg
Salt and freshly ground black pepper

1 Fry (sauté) the onion in the butter, stirring until a rich golden brown, about 5–6 minutes.

2 Wash the spinach well and discard any thick stalks. Tear into pieces, shaking off excess moisture. Place in a saucepan with no extra water. Cover and cook over a moderate heat for about 5 minutes until tender, shaking the pan occasionally.

3 Remove the lid and boil rapidly for 1 minute to evaporate any moisture, stirring.

4 Stir in the cream, nutmeg and a little salt and pepper and cook, stirring for 1 minute. Spoon into a serving dish and top with the buttery onions. Serve hot.

Braised Leeks

SERVES 2

2 leeks, sliced
20 g/1½ oz/4 tsp butter
Good pinch of ground coriander (cilantro)
Salt and freshly ground black pepper

1 Cook the leeks in the butter in a saucepan over a moderate heat for 3 minutes, stirring.

2 Add just enough water to part-cover the leeks, bring to the boil, reduce the heat and cook for 4–5 minutes until tender. Stir once or twice during cooking.

3 Boil rapidly for 1 minute to reduce the liquid. Season with the coriander and some salt and pepper and serve.

Celery and Carrot Pot

SERVES 2

3 celery sticks, sliced
3 carrots, sliced
1 onion, sliced
15 g/½ oz/1 tbsp butter
30 ml/2 tbsp sunflower oil
2.5 ml/½ tsp dried oregano
1 vegetable stock cube
150 ml/¼ pt/⅔ cup boiling water

1 Fry (sauté) the celery, carrots and onion in the butter and oil for 3 minutes, stirring.

2 Blend the oregano and vegetable stock cube with the water, then pour into the pan.

3 Part-cover and cook for 8 minutes. Remove the lid and cook for 3–4 minutes more until the vegetables are tender and nearly all the liquid has evaporated. Serve hot.

Broccoli and Cauliflower Stir-fry

SERVES 2–4

½ onion, finely chopped
30 ml/2 tbsp olive oil
½ small cauliflower, cut into florets
175 g/6 oz broccoli, cut into florets
5 ml/1 tsp coriander (cilantro) seeds, crushed
Salt and freshly ground black pepper
15 g/½ oz/1 tbsp butter
1 small garlic clove, crushed

1 Fry (sauté) the onion in the oil in a large frying pan (skillet) or wok.

2 Add the cauliflower and broccoli and fry for 2 minutes.

3 Add the crushed coriander seeds and continue frying, stirring for 5 minutes. Season.

4 Add the butter and garlic and cook for a further 2 minutes until golden but still crunchy.

Puréed Carrots and Peas

SERVES 2

2 large carrots
100 g/4 oz shelled peas
30 ml/2 tbsp single (light) cream
Salt and freshly ground black pepper
1.5 ml/¼ tsp dried mint
25 g/1 oz/2 tbsp butter

1 Cook the carrots and peas separately in lightly salted boiling water until tender. Drain, reserving the pea cooking water.

2 Purée the vegetables separately in a blender. Return to their cooking saucepans.

3 Beat the cream into the carrots and season with pepper. Reheat.

4 Add the mint to the peas and beat in the butter. Moisten, if necessary, with a little of the cooking water to give a smooth purée. Reheat before serving.

Nutty Cauliflower

SERVES 2

½ cauliflower, separated into florets
Salt and freshly ground black pepper
40 g/1½ oz/3 tbsp butter
30 ml/2 tbsp flaked almonds

1 Cook the cauliflower in boiling, lightly salted water until tender. Drain and place in a warm serving dish.

2 Dust with freshly ground black pepper. Keep warm.

3 Melt the butter and fry (sauté) the almonds until golden. Pour immediately over the cauliflower and serve.

Broccoli with Hazelnut Sauce

SERVES 2

225 g/8 oz broccoli, cut into florets
150 ml/¼ pt/⅔ cup vegetable stock
50 g/2 oz/½ cup ground hazelnuts
Pinch of salt
Knob of butter
To garnish:
A few toasted chopped hazelnuts

1 Cook the broccoli in the stock until just tender.

2 Lift out with a draining spoon and transfer to a warm serving dish.

3 Whisk in the ground nuts, a pinch of salt and the butter. Thin with a little water if necessary.

4 Spoon over the broccoli and flash under a hot grill (broiler) to glaze.

Fruity Red Cabbage

SERVES 2

This recipe must be served with a protein-rich meal.

½ small red cabbage (about 350 g/12 oz), shredded
1 onion, sliced
75 ml/5 tbsp apple juice
10 ml/2 tsp caraway seeds
Salt and freshly ground black pepper
1 eating (dessert) apple, diced
50 g/2 oz black grapes, halved and seeded (pitted)

1 Mix the cabbage with the onion, apple juice, caraway seeds and a little salt and pepper in a saucepan.

2 Bring to the boil, reduce the heat, cover and cook over a very gentle heat for 40 minutes or until the cabbage is tender, stirring frequently.

3 Stir in the apple and grapes and serve.

Red Slaw with Walnuts

SERVES 2

¼ small red cabbage, coarsely grated
½ small red onion, sliced
2 beetroot (red beets), coarsely grated
50 g/2 oz/½ cup walnuts, roughly chopped
45 ml/3 tbsp soured (dairy sour) cream
Salt and freshly ground black pepper
To garnish:
Snipped chives

1 Mix all the ingredients together in a bowl.

2 Garnish with chives and chill before serving.

Sesame Bean Sprout Salad

SERVES 2

1 green (bell) pepper, cut into short, thin strips
1 carrot, cut in short, thin strips
2 spring onions (scallions), chopped
2 tomatoes, roughly chopped
100 g/4 oz bean sprouts
25 g/1 oz/¼ cup sesame seeds
10 ml/2 tsp sesame oil
10 ml/2 tsp sunflower oil
Salt and freshly ground black pepper
10 ml/2 tsp soy sauce (if serving as
    part of a protein meal)

1 Mix the vegetables together in a bowl.

2 Dry-fry the sesame seeds in a frying pan (skillet) until lightly browned. Add to the salad.

3 Drizzle with the oils and season to taste. Toss.

4 Sprinkle with soy sauce if serving as part of a protein meal, otherwise omit.

Peasant Mixed Salad

SERVES 2

¼ **cos (romaine) lettuce**
1 red onion, sliced into rings
¼ **cucumber, diced**
1 carrot, grated
1 turnip, grated
Handful of sunflower seeds
2 ripe tomatoes, skinned and very finely chopped
15 ml/1 tbsp olive oil
1.5 ml/¼ tsp mustard
Freshly ground black pepper

1 Tear the lettuce into pieces and place in a bowl with the onion, cucumber, carrot, turnip and sunflower seeds.

2 Whisk the remaining ingredients thoroughly together and add to the bowl.

3 Toss and serve.

Rainbow Salad

SERVES 2

1 each green, red and yellow (bell) peppers,
  cut in thin strips
1 beetroot (red beet), cut into thin strips
¼ **cucumber, cut into thin strips**
1 carrot, cut into thin strips
2 tomatoes, chopped
4 lettuce leaves, shredded
30 ml/2 tbsp olive oil
15 ml/1 tbsp chopped parsley
15 ml/1 tbsp chopped mint
1 garlic clove, crushed

1 Arrange all the vegetables attractively on a serving platter.

2 Warm the oil, stir in the herbs and garlic and drizzle over. Serve straight away.

Warm Courgette and Carrot Salad

SERVES 2

2 large carrots, grated
2 courgettes (zucchini), grated
Salt and freshly ground black pepper
30 ml/2 tbsp olive oil
15 g/½ oz/1 tbsp butter
30 ml/2 tbsp black mustard seeds

1 Mix the grated vegetables in a salad bowl. Season with salt and pepper.

2 Heat the oil and butter in a frying pan (skillet) and fry (sauté) the mustard seeds until they begin to 'pop'.

3 Pour the contents of the pan over the vegetables, toss quickly and serve straight away.

Village Garden Salad

SERVES 2

½ round lettuce
2 celery sticks, sliced
50 g/2 oz/½ cup walnut halves
6 radishes, sliced
50 g/2 oz fresh shelled peas
30 ml/2 tbsp home-made mayonnaise
   (see Russian Salad Deluxe page 110)
Freshly ground black pepper
To garnish:
Sprig of parsley

1 Separate the leaves and use to line two serving bowls.

2 Mix the celery, walnuts, radishes and peas with the mayonnaise. Pile on to the lettuce and garnish each with a sprig of parsley.

Nutty Slaw

SERVES 2

¼ small white cabbage, finely shredded
1 carrot, coarsely grated
1 celery stick, chopped
¼ onion, grated
50 g/2 oz/½ cup Dry-roasted Nuts (see page 156)
30 ml/2 tbsp home-made mayonnaise
  (see Russian Salad Deluxe page 110)
15 ml/1 tbsp buttermilk
Good pinch of cayenne
Freshly ground black pepper
To garnish:
Chopped parsley

1 Mix the cabbage, carrot, celery and onion in a bowl with the peanuts.

2 Blend the mayonnaise with the buttermilk and stir in. Season with cayenne and freshly ground black pepper. Garnish with parsley before serving.

Fennel and Hazelnut Crunch

SERVES 2

45 ml/3 tbsp whole hazelnuts
15 ml/½ oz/1 tbsp butter
1 large or 2 small heads of fennel
45 ml/3 tbsp olive oil
Salt and freshly ground black pepper
6 cherry tomatoes, halved

1 Fry (sauté) the hazelnuts in the butter until golden brown. Drain on kitchen paper.

2 Trim off any damaged outer stalks from the fennel then slice thinly across the bulbs.

3 Lay on two flat plates. Drizzle with olive oil and season with salt and pepper.

4 Scatter the hazelnuts over and add the halved cherry tomatoes before serving.

Athena Salad

SERVES 2

¼ iceberg lettuce, shredded
2 red (bell) peppers, quartered
2 ripe tomatoes, sliced
½ red onion, sliced into rings
8 stuffed olives
Coarse sea salt
Freshly ground black pepper
15 ml/1 tbsp olive oil

1 Put the shredded lettuce on two serving plates.

2 Grill (broil) the peppers until tender and slightly blackened. Lay on the lettuce.

3 Arrange the tomato slices around and scatter the onion rings and olives over.

4 Sprinkle with coarse sea salt and freshly ground black pepper.

5 Drizzle the oil over and serve.

Cooling Cucumber

SERVES 2

½ cucumber, diced
150 ml/¼ pt/⅔ cup crème fraîche
Grated rind of 1 lime
5 ml/1 tsp dried mint
Salt and freshly ground black pepper

1 Mix the cucumber with the crème fraîche, lime rind and mint and season to taste.

2 Chill until ready to serve.

Mixed Green Salad

SERVES 2

1 little gem lettuce
1 bunch of watercress
5 cm/2 in piece of cucumber, sliced
1 green (bell) pepper, sliced
1 avocado, sliced
Dressing (optional):
30 ml/2 tbsp olive oil
Salt and freshly ground black pepper
2.5 ml/½ tsp mustard
5 ml/1 tsp chopped parsley
5 ml/1 tsp chopped oregano
1 stalk of lemon grass, finely chopped

1 Separate the lettuce into leaves, tear into pieces and place in a salad bowl.

2 Discard any feathery stalks from the watercress and add to the bowl.

3 Add the cucumber, pepper and avocado.

4 Whisk the dressing ingredients together and drizzle over just before serving if using.

Tomato and Onion Salad

SERVES 2

4 ripe tomatoes, sliced
1 small onion, finely chopped
15 ml/1 tbsp chopped parsley
15 ml/1 tbsp olive oil
Salt and freshly ground black pepper

1 Arrange the tomato slices in a shallow serving dish.

2 Sprinkle the onion and parsley over.

3 Drizzle with the oil and sprinkle with salt and pepper. Leave to stand for 1 hour, if possible, before serving.

Green Bean and Tomato Salad

SERVES 2

**175 g/6 oz dwarf green beans, topped and tailed
but left whole
1 small onion, finely chopped
3 tomatoes, skinned and chopped
15 ml/1 tbsp chopped parsley or coriander
(cilantro)
15 ml/1 tbsp olive oil
Freshly ground black pepper**

1 Cook the beans in boiling, lightly salted water until just tender. Drain, rinse with cold water and drain again.

2 Lay all the same way in a shallow oblong dish.

3 Mix the onion and tomatoes together with the herbs and spoon over the beans. Drizzle with olive oil and add a good grinding of pepper.

4 Chill for at least 1 hour before serving.

Tomato, Chive and Carrot Salad

SERVES 2

**2 beefsteak tomatoes
3 carrots, grated
30 ml/2 tbsp snipped chives
15 ml/1 tbsp sesame seeds
15 ml/1 tbsp olive oil
Salt and pepper**

1 Cut a slice off the top of each tomato and scoop out the seeds.

2 Mix the carrots and chives in a bowl.

3 Fry the sesame seeds in the oil briefly to brown. Pour over the carrots with some salt and pepper and toss.

4 Pile into the tomatoes and serve.

Avocado and Bean Sprout Salad

SERVES 2

100 g/4 oz bean sprouts
50 g/2 oz/½ cup walnuts, roughly chopped
1 avocado, diced
1 spring onion (scallion), finely chopped
1 red (bell) pepper, chopped
Dressing:
2 ripe tomatoes
15 ml/1 tbsp sunflower oil
5 ml/1 tsp Chinese five spice powder
Freshly ground black pepper

1 Mix the salad ingredients together and divide between two bowls.

2 Make the dressing. Purée the tomato with the oil and five spice powder. Season with pepper. Spoon over the salad and serve.

Carrot, Beetroot and Celeriac Salad

SERVES 2

2 large carrots, coarsely grated
½ head of celeriac (celery root), coarsely grated
2 spring onions (scallions), chopped
45 ml/3 tbsp crème fraîche
Salt and freshly ground black pepper
30 ml/2 tbsp sunflower seeds
4 beetroot (red beets), diced
To garnish:
Chopped coriander (cilantro) or parsley

1 Mix the carrots, celeriac and spring onions together in a bowl.

2 Add the crème fraîche and seasoning to taste and toss well.

3 Divide between two serving plates. Shape into nests and sprinkle with sunflower seeds. Pile the beetroot in the centre, garnish with coriander or parsley and serve straight away.

Italian Salad

SERVES 2

¼ small iceberg lettuce
¼ head of celeriac (celery root), grated
2 carrots, grated
2 tomatoes, cut in wedges
8 green olives
½ small onion, sliced into thin rings
Dressing:
1 large ripe tomato, roughly chopped
15 ml/1 tbsp olive oil
15 ml/1 tbsp cold water
2 basil leaves, chopped
Salt and freshly ground black pepper

1 Tear the lettuce into pieces and arrange on two serving plates.

2 Pile the grated vegetables on top and arrange the tomato wedges around.

3 Scatter the olives and onion rings over.

4 Purée all the dressing ingredients in a blender. Sieve (strain), if liked, and drizzle over the salads. Dust with a little more black pepper before serving.

Mixed Leaf Salad

Use any combination of leaves: rocket, lamb's tongue, lollo rosso, little gem, radicchio, young spinach and any fresh, torn herbs like basil, coriander (cilantro), parsley.

Dress with a little olive oil, salt and pepper and puréed fresh tomato to serve with a neutral or carbohydrate meal or substitute lemon juice for the tomato if serving with a protein meal.

SNACKS

All these snacks are ideal for 'bridging the gap' between meals. But if you're trying to lose a lot of weight stick to fruit or raw vegetables for your nibbles and only when genuinely hungry.

PROTEIN-RICH

Enjoy these in the mornings for special treats as a change from a piece of fruit .

Fruity Yoghurt Shake

SERVES 1

100 g/4 oz ripe strawberries, or 1 peeled and
   stoned (pitted) ripe peach or nectarine
75 ml/5 tbsp thick, plain yoghurt
150 ml/¼ pt/⅔ cup ice cold milk

1 Purée the fruit in a blender.

2 Add the yoghurt and milk and run the machine until the mixture is frothy.

3 Pour into a glass and serve.

Fresh Strawberry Milkshake

SERVES 1

100 g/4 oz ripe strawberries
150 ml/¼ pt/⅓ cup milk (or half milk, half single
   (light) cream)
4 ice cubes

1 Put all the ingredients in a blender and run the machine until the fruit is puréed.

2 Pour into a glass and serve.

Fresh Apricot Yoghurt

SERVES 1

3 fresh apricots
30 ml/2 tbsp apple juice
150 ml/¼ pt/⅔ cup thick, plain yoghurt

1 Skin the apricots and discard the stones (pits).

2 Purée with the apple juice in a blender. Spoon into a glass dish and top with the yoghurt.

Vanilla Yoghurt Shake

SERVES 1

150 ml/¼ pt/⅔ mild, thick, plain yoghurt
5 ml/1 tsp natural vanilla essence (extract)
150 ml/¼ pt/⅔ cup apple juice

1 Put all the ingredients in a container, seal and shake thoroughly until well blended.

2 Pour into a tall glass and serve straight away.

Cheese-stuffed Celery

SERVES 1

2 celery sticks
25 g/1 oz/2 tbsp low-fat soft cheese

1 Trim the celery then fill the groove in each stick with the cheese, spreading it in with a knife.

2 Cut into short pieces and serve.

Fennel-Cheese Boats

SERVES 1

25 g/1 oz/¼ cup Cheddar cheese, grated
15 g/½ oz/1 tbsp butter
10 ml/2 tsp fennel seeds, lightly crushed
2 celery sticks

1 Mash the cheese and butter together with the fennel seeds.

2 Spread in the celery sticks.

3 Cut into short lengths and serve.

Blackcurrant Cooler

SERVES 1

100g/4 oz blackcurrants
Apple juice
Crushed ice
Sprig of mint

1 Purée the blackcurrants in a blender.

2 With the machine still running, add as much apple juice as liked (I use about 200 ml/7 fl oz/scant 1 cup) to make a palatable drink.

3 Strain over crushed ice in a tall glass and garnish with a sprig of mint.

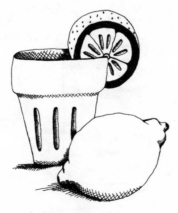

Tomato Pick-me-up

SERVES 1

2 ripe tomatoes, quartered
45 ml/3 tbsp freshly squeezed orange juice
Pinch of chilli powder
Good dash of soy sauce
Crushed ice

1 Purée the tomatoes in a blender with the orange juice and chilli powder. Add soy sauce to taste.

2 Strain over crushed ice into a glass and serve.

Yoghurt with Crushed Berries

SERVES 1

50 g/2 oz strawberries
50 g/2 oz raspberries
Grated rind and juice of 1 clementine
150 ml/¼ pt/⅔ cup thick, plain yoghurt

1 Mash the strawberries and raspberries lightly and stir in the clementine rind and juice.

2 Fold in the yoghurt and chill for at least 1 hour (if possible) before serving.

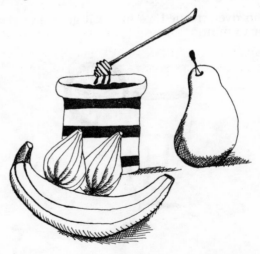

CARBOHYDRATE-RICH

These are ideal for tea-time treats – go easy on the butter!

Banana Tea Bread

MAKES 1 LOAF

2 ripe bananas
5 ml/1 tsp bicarbonate of soda (baking soda)
45 ml/3 tbsp clear honey
50 g/2 oz/¼ cup butter
275 g/10 oz/2½ cups wholemeal self-raising
   (self-rising) flour
1 egg yolk
45 ml/3 tbsp water
To serve:
Scraping of butter

1 Put the bananas, bicarbonate of soda, honey and butter in a food processor and blend until smooth.

2 Add the flour, egg yolk and water and blend in until just mixed.

3 Turn into a greased 900 g/2 lb loaf tin (pan) and bake in a preheated oven at 180°C/350°F/gas mark 4 for about 50 minutes–1 hour until risen, golden and firm to the touch.

4 Leave to cool slightly in the tin then turn out on to a wire rack to cool. Serve sliced with a scraping of butter.

Fruit Scones

MAKES 6

225 g/8 oz/2 cups wholemeal self-raising
  (self-rising) flour
7.5 ml/1½ tsp baking powder
50 g/2 oz/¼ cup butter
75 g/3 oz/½ cup sultanas (golden raisins)
Buttermilk
To serve:
Scraping of butter

1 Mix the flour with the baking powder in a bowl.

2 Rub in the butter.

3 Stir in the sultanas and mix with enough buttermilk to form a soft but not sticky dough.

4 Shape into a round about 2 cm/¾ in thick.

5 Cut into scones using a fluted 6 cm/2½ in cutter.

6 Place on a lightly greased baking sheet and brush with a little extra buttermilk to glaze. Bake in a preheated oven at 220°C/425°F/gas mark 7 for about 15 minutes or until risen and the bases sound hollow when tapped.

7 Cool on a wire rack, serve split and spread with a scraping of butter.

Italian Open Sandwich

SERVES 1

15 ml/1 tbsp Mascarpone cheese
4 black olives, stoned (pitted) and chopped
1 slice wholemeal bread
1 ripe tomato, sliced
4 basil leaves, torn
Freshly ground black pepper

1 Mash the cheese with the olives and spread over the bread. Cut in half.

2 Arrange the tomato slices over and scatter with the basil.

3 Add a good grinding of pepper and serve.

Banana and Raisin Sandwich

Butter
4 slices of wholemeal bread
50 g/2 oz/⅓ cup raisins
1 large banana
Pinch of ground cinnamon

1 Lightly butter the bread.

2 Put the raisins in a bowl and snip with scissors to chop fairly finely.

3 Add the banana and mash well with a fork until mixed together thoroughly.

4 Spread over two slices of the bread and top with the remaining slices. Cut into triangles and serve.

Cucumber and Cress Butter Sandwiches

45 ml/3 tbsp cress (or mustard and cress)
25 g/1 oz/2 tbsp butter
4 thin slices of wholemeal bread
2.5 cm/1 in piece of cucumber, thinly sliced
Freshly ground black pepper

1 Put the cress into a bowl and snip with scissors to chop.

2 Add the butter and mash together well.

3 Spread over the slices of bread.

4 Top two slices with cucumber and season with pepper. Top with the remaining slices and cut into triangles.

Sesame Butter and Cress Pinwheels

SERVES 1

1 thin slice of wholemeal bread, crusts removed
Home-made Sesame Butter (see page 156)
Cress
Freshly ground black pepper

1 Spread the bread with the Sesame Butter and sprinkle thickly with cress.

2 Roll up and wrap in greaseproof (waxed) paper. Chill, if time.

3 Unwrap and cut into slices. Serve.

Tomato and Chive Sandwich

SERVES 1

15 g/½ oz/1 tbsp butter
15 ml/1 tbsp snipped chives
2 thin slices wholemeal bread
1 tomato, sliced
Freshly ground black pepper

1 Mash the butter with the chives and spread on the bread.

2 Top one slice with the tomato and sprinkle with black pepper.

3 Top with the second slice and cut into quarters.

Salad Sandwich

SERVES 1

Butter
2 thin slices of wholemeal bread
1 lettuce leaf
4 thin slices of cucumber
1 radish, sliced
1 tomato, sliced
Freshly ground black pepper

1 Butter the bread thinly.

2 Lay the lettuce leaf on one slice and top with the remaining salad ingredients.

3 Dust with black pepper and top with the second slice of bread. Press down firmly but gently. Cut into triangles.

Cucumber and Mascarpone Sandwich

SERVES 1

2 slices of wholemeal bread
30 ml/2 tbsp Mascarpone cheese
4 slices of cucumber
Good pinch dried dill (dill weed)
Freshly ground black pepper

1 Spread the bread with the cheese.

2 Top with the cucumber then sprinkle with dill and pepper.

3 Cover with the second slice of bread and cut into quarters.

Chewy Pear Bars

MAKES 15

175 ml/6 fl oz/¾ cup single (light) cream
60 ml/4 tbsp thick honey
100 g/4 oz/½ cup butter
50 g/2 oz/⅓ cup sultanas (golden raisins)
50 g/2 oz/⅓ cup raisins
225 g/8 oz ready-to-eat dried pears, chopped
100 g/4 oz/1 cup desiccated (shredded) coconut
225 g/8 oz/2 cups rolled oats

1 Heat the cream with the honey and butter in a saucepan until the butter melts.

2 Stir in the remaining ingredients.

3 Press into a 28x18 cm/11x7 in shallow baking tin (pan).

4 Cover with clingfilm (plastic wrap) and chill overnight before cutting into bars.

Cinnamon Toast

SERVES 2

1 egg yolk
30 ml/2 tbsp buttermilk
15 ml/1 tbsp water
15 ml/1 tbsp clear honey
2 slices of wholemeal bread, crusts removed
15 g/½ oz/1 tbsp butter
15 ml/1 tbsp sunflower oil
Ground cinnamon

1 Beat the egg yolk with the buttermilk, water and honey until well blended.

2 Soak the bread completely in the mixture.

3 Heat the butter and oil in a frying pan (skillet) and fry (sauté) the bread on each side until golden brown.

4 Sprinkle with cinnamon and serve cut into triangles.

Jumbo Digestive Biscuits

MAKES ABOUT 12

225 g/8 oz/2 cups wholemeal flour
1.5 ml/¼ tsp salt
2.5 ml/½ tsp bicarbonate of soda (baking soda)
75 g/3 oz/⅓ cup butter
45 ml/3 tbsp thick honey
1 egg yolk
45 ml/3 tbsp buttermilk

1 Mix the flour, salt and bicarbonate of soda in a bowl.

2 Rub in the butter then work in the honey, egg yolk and enough buttermilk to form a firm dough.

3 Knead gently on a lightly floured surface. Roll out to about 5 mm/¼ in thick and cut into large biscuits (cookies) using a 7.5 cm/3 in cutter.

4 Transfer to a lightly greased baking sheet and prick attractively with a fork. Bake in a preheated oven at 190°C/375°F/gas mark 5 for about 15 minutes or until golden.

5 Leave to cool for 10 minutes then transfer to a wire rack to cool completely. Store in an airtight tin.

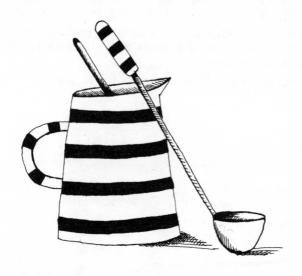

Singin' Hinny

SERVES 6

350 g/12 oz/3 cups wholemeal self-raising
(self-rising) flour
10 ml/2 tsp baking powder
2.5 ml/½ tsp salt
50 g/2 oz/¼ cup butter
100 g/4 oz/⅔ cup currants
150 ml/¼ pt/⅔ cup buttermilk
A little sunflower oil for greasing
To serve:
Butter

1 Mix the flour, baking powder and salt together in a bowl.

2 Add the butter and rub in with the fingertips. Stir in the currants.

3 Mix with enough buttermilk to form a soft but not sticky dough.

4 Knead gently on a lightly floured surface. Pat out to a round about 1 cm/½ in thick or a little thinner.

5 Lightly oil a frying pan (skillet). Heat the pan over a gentle heat then add the dough and cook gently for about 6 minutes until golden underneath – it will 'sing' as it sizzles and cooks!

6 Turn over with a fish slice and continue cooking until brown underneath and cooked through. Slide out of the pan on to a plate.

7 Cut into wedges, split in half and butter lightly.

Dropped Scones

MAKES ABOUT 12

100 g/4 oz/1 cup wholemeal self-raising
  (self-rising) flour
Pinch of salt
15 ml/1 tbsp clear honey
1 egg yolk
30 ml/2 tbsp water
150 ml/¼ pt/⅔ cup buttermilk
A little oil for greasing

1 Mix the flour and salt together in a bowl.

2 Mix the honey, egg yolk and water together and beat into the flour until smooth.

3 Stir in the buttermilk.

4 Heat a heavy-based frying pan (skillet) and grease lightly. Drop spoonfuls of the mixture into the hot pan and cook until golden brown underneath (about 2 minutes). Flip over with a fish slice and cook the other sides. Keep warm in a napkin while cooking the remainder.

Carrot Cake

SERVES 6–8

225 g/8 oz/2 cups wholemeal self-raising
  (self-rising) flour
15 ml/1 tbsp baking powder
150 g/5 oz/⅔ cup butter
60 ml/4 tbsp thick honey
2 large carrots, grated
5 ml/1 tsp mixed (apple pie) spice

1 Mix the flour and baking powder.

2 Melt the butter and honey and stir in with the carrots and spice.

3 Turn into a greased 450 g/1 lb loaf tin (pan) and bake in a preheated oven at 160°C/325°F/gas mark 3 for about 1 hour until risen, golden and a skewer inserted in the centre comes out clean. Serve cut into slices.

Teacup Cake

SERVES 8

Use the same cup to measure each ingredient.

½ cup butter
1 cup currants
½ cup sultanas (golden raisins)
½ cup chopped mixed nuts
1 cup thick honey
1 cup cold decaffeinated tea
5 ml/1 tsp dried mint
2 cups wholemeal self-raising (self-rising) flour

1 Put all the ingredients except the flour in a saucepan and heat gently, stirring until the butter melts. Bring to the boil and simmer for 3 minutes.

2 Leave to cool slightly then stir in the flour.

3 Turn into a greased 900 g/2 lb loaf tin (pan).

4 Bake immediately in a preheated oven at 180°C/350°F/gas mark 4 for about 50 minutes until well risen, golden and a skewer inserted in the centre comes out clean.

5 Cool slightly then turn out of the tin and leave to cool on a wire rack. Serve sliced.

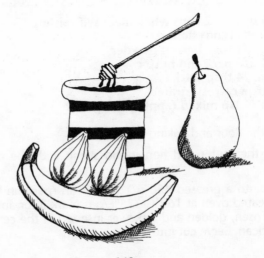

Vitality Scones

MAKES 8

225 g/8 oz/2 cups wholemeal self-raising
  (self-rising) flour
10 ml/2 tsp baking powder
15 ml/1 tbsp bran
Pinch of salt
50 g/2 oz/¼ cup butter
45 ml/3 tbsp clear honey
2 whole dried bananas, chopped
25 g/1 oz/1 tbsp sultanas (golden raisins)
1 egg yolk
30 ml/2 tbsp water
45 ml/3 tbsp crème fraîche
To serve:
Butter

1 Mix the flour and baking powder together in a bowl with the bran and salt.

2 Rub in the butter.

3 Stir in the honey and fruit.

4 Blend the egg yolk with the water and crème fraîche, add to the bowl and mix to form a firm dough.

5 Knead into a ball and pat out to a round about 2 cm/¾ in thick.

6 Cut into rounds using a 6.5 cm/2½ in cutter.

7 Place on a greased baking sheet and bake in a preheated oven at 220°C/425°F/gas mark 7 for about 10–15 minutes until well risen and golden and the bases sound hollow when tapped. Serve split and lightly buttered.

Carob Chews

MAKES 15

30 ml/2 tbsp thick honey
30 ml/2 tbsp unrefined black molasses
75 g/3 oz/⅓ cup butter
225 g/8 oz/2 cups rolled oats
45 ml/3 tbsp carob powder
5 ml/1 tsp natural vanilla essence (extract)
25 g/1 oz/¼ cup walnuts, chopped
50 g/2 oz/⅓ cup sultanas (golden raisins) chopped

1 Put the honey, molasses and butter in a large pan and heat until the butter melts.

2 Stir in the remaining ingredients. Press into a greased, shallow baking tin (pan) and chill until firm.

3 Cut into bars and store in an airtight container in the fridge.

Branflake Cakes

MAKES ABOUT 16

75 g/3 oz/⅓ cup butter
75 ml/5 tbsp thick honey
45 ml/3 tbsp carob powder
100 g/4 oz/4 cups natural bran flakes
    (without added sugar)

1 Melt the butter, honey and carob powder.

2 Stir in the flakes until completely coated.

3 Spoon into paper cake cases (cupcake papers) and chill until set.

DESSERTS

Make sure you only serve these as part of a protein-rich meal. If you're trying to lose weight have low-fat yoghurt rather than cream as an accompaniment to fresh fruit. A fresh fruit salad is a good dessert for any protein-rich meal.

Fresh Fruit Salad

SERVES 2

150 ml/¼ pt/⅔ cup apple juice
1 red eating (dessert) apple, diced
1 orange, pith and peel removed and segmented
1 kiwi fruit, sliced
1 nectarine, sliced

1 Pour the apple juice into a bowl.

2 Add the prepared fruits and chill, preferably for 2 hours, to allow the flavours to develop before serving.

Zabaglione

SERVES 2

2 egg yolks
90 ml/6 tbsp sweet sherry or marsala wine

1 Put the egg yolks and sherry in a bowl over a pan of gently simmering water.

2 Whisk with an electric beater until thick and foamy.

3 Turn into two stemmed glasses and serve straight away.

Strawberry Yoghurt Brûlé

SERVES 2

175 g/6 oz strawberries, sliced
75 ml/5 tbsp thick, plain yoghurt
Few drops of natural vanilla essence (extract)
75 ml/5 tbsp double (heavy) cream
30 ml/2 tbsp sesame seeds

1 Put half the strawberries in two small, flameproof dishes. Mash the remainder.

2 Whip the yoghurt, vanilla and cream together until stiff. Fold in the mashed strawberries. Spread over the sliced strawberries and chill.

3 Sprinkle the tops with sesame seeds to coat completely.

4 Place under a hot grill (broiler) until the sesame seeds turn golden.

5 Serve straight away.

Spiced Oranges

SERVES 2

4 oranges
90 ml/6 tbsp apple juice
2.5 ml/½ tsp mixed (apple pie) spice
5 ml/1 tsp lemon juice

1 Peel all the rind and pith from the oranges. Cut into slices then hold together with cocktail sticks (toothpicks). Place in a dish and pour any juice over.

2 Simmer the apple juice with the spice and lemon juice for 3 minutes. Pour over the oranges and leave until cold.

Mixed Berries with Crème Fraîche

SERVES 2

50 g/2 oz raspberries
50 g/2 oz strawberries
50 g/2 oz cultivated blackberries
50 g/2 oz blueberries
45 ml/3 tbsp crème fraîche
2.5 ml/½ tsp natural vanilla essence (extract)

1 Arrange all the berries attractively on two serving plates.

2 Mix the crème fraîche with the vanilla essence and put a large spoonful on each plate.

Lemon Velvet

SERVES 2

10 ml/2 tsp gelatine (or vegetarian equivalent)
300 ml/½ pt/1¼ cups pineapple juice
1 lemon
150 ml/¼ pt/⅔ cup double (heavy) cream,
   whipped
To decorate:
Sprig of mint

1 Dissolve the gelatine in a little of the pineapple juice according to packet directions.

2 Stir in the remaining juice.

3 Grate the lemon rind and add. Squeeze the juice. Add as much as you like to give a good lemony flavour but not too sour.

4 Chill until the consistency of egg white.

5 Gradually whisk in the cream, transfer to two serving dishes and chill until set. Decorate each with a sprig of mint.

Peach Melba

SERVES 2

2 ripe peaches
45 ml/3 tbsp low-fat soft cheese
Grated rind and juice of 1 orange
100 g/4 oz raspberries

1 Remove the skins from the peaches, cut in halves and remove the stones (pits).

2 Mash the cheese with the orange rind. Sandwich the peaches back together with the flavoured cheese.

3 Place in two glass dishes.

4 Purée the raspberries with the orange juice. Pass through a sieve (strainer) to remove the seeds then spoon over the peaches.

Pineapple with Coconut

SERVES 2

2 thick slices of fresh pineapple, peeled
60 ml/4 tbsp desiccated (shredded) coconut
A little crème fraîche (optional)

1 Cut out any thick central core from the pineapple and pat the flesh dry on kitchen paper.

2 Toast the coconut in a dry frying pan (skillet) until golden, stirring.

3 Press the pineapple into the coconut on both sides until well coated.

4 Place on serving plates and serve straight away with a little crème fraîche spooned into the centre, if liked.

Jaffa Apples

SERVES 2

1 large orange
150 ml/¼ pt/⅔ cup apple juice
2 eating (dessert) apples, sliced

1 Cut the rind off the orange and cut into thin strips. Boil in the apple juice for 5 minutes until tender. Remove the rind with a draining spoon and reserve.

2 Cut off the pith from the orange then divide into segments between the membranes.

3 Place the fruit in a bowl with the apple slices. Pour over the hot apple juice and leave to cool. Scatter the orange rind over and chill until ready to serve.

Fresh Blackberry and Apple Compote

SERVES 2

150 ml/¼ pt/⅔ cup apple juice
2 eating (dessert) apples, grated
100 g/4 oz cultivated sweet, ripe blackberries

1 Mix the apple juice with the grated apples and blackberries.

2 Cover and chill for at least 3 hours or preferably overnight to allow the flavours to develop.

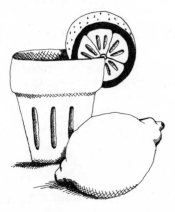

Cider Syllabub

SERVES 2

150 ml/¼ pt/⅔ cup double (heavy) cream
Grated rind and juice of ½ lemon
45 ml/3 tbsp sweet cider

1 Whip the cream until just peaking.

2 Gently whisk the lemon rind, juice and the cider into the cream.

3 Spoon into two glasses and chill for at least 2 hours. The mixture may separate into a creamy layer with the lemony juice underneath.

Fresh Orange Jelly

SERVES 2

Grated rind and juice of 4 large oranges
A little apple juice
10 ml/2 tsp gelatine (or vegetarian equivalent)

1 Put the orange rind and juice in a measuring jug and make up to 300 ml/½ pt with apple juice.

2 Dissolve the gelatine in a little of the liquid according to packet directions. Stir in the remaining juice.

3 Pour into two glasses and chill until set.

CARBOHYDRATE-RICH

Serve these after a carbohydrate-rich main course.

Fried Fruity Sandwich

SERVES 2

2 slices of wholemeal bread, buttered lightly on
   both sides
30 ml/2 tbsp raisins
2 dried figs, finely chopped
Ground cinnamon
To serve:
Crème fraîche (optional)

1 Sandwich the bread with the raisins, figs and a dusting of cinnamon. Press firmly together.

2 Fry (sauté) until golden brown underneath, pressing down with a fish slice.

3 Carefully turn over and fry the other side until golden.

4 Cut in half and serve with a little crème fraîche, if liked.

Dried Fruit Compote

SERVES 2

225 g/8 oz mixed dried figs, prunes and pears
300 ml/½ pt/1¼ cups water
2.5 ml/1 in piece of cinnamon stick

1 Soak the salad in the water for at least 4 hours or preferably overnight.

2 Add the cinnamon stick, bring to the boil, reduce the heat, cover and simmer gently for 30 minutes until the fruit is tender.

3 Remove the cinnamon stick and serve hot or chilled.

Date Slices

MAKES 16

350 g/12 oz/3 cups wholemeal flour
175 g/6 oz butter
60 ml/4 tbsp clear honey
1 egg yolk
45 ml/3 tbsp water
250 g/9 oz/1 block, stoned (pitted) dates
5 ml/1 tsp mixed (apple pie) spice

1 Put the flour in a bowl. Add the butter and rub in with the fingertips until the mixture resembles breadcrumbs.

2 Blend the honey with the egg yolk and water and mix to form a firm dough, adding a little more water if necessary.

3 Knead gently, cut in half and press one half to a rectangle to line an 18x28cm/7x11 in Swiss roll tin (jelly roll pan).

4 Spread the dates over and sprinkle with the mixed spice.

5 Roll out the remaining dough and lay over the dates. It may crack but just gently press together again. Crimp the edges between the finger and thumb.

6 Cook in a preheated oven at 180°C/350°F/gas mark 4 for about 40 minutes until golden. Leave to cool in the tin then cut into 16 bars. Store in an airtight tin.

Banana Cheese

SERVES 2

2 ripe bananas
Grated rind of ½ lime
75 g/3 oz/⅓ cup Mascarpone cheese
30 ml/2 tbsp single (light) cream

1 Mash the bananas thoroughly with the lime rind.

2 Beat the Mascarpone cheese with the cream until smooth, then beat into the bananas.

3 Spoon into small glass dishes and serve chilled.

Creamy Rice Pudding

SERVES 4

50 g/2 oz/¼ cup brown round grain (pudding) rice
30 ml/2 tbsp clear honey
300 ml/½ pt/1¼ cups water
300 ml/½ pt/1¼ cups double (heavy) cream
A little grated nutmeg
Knob of butter

1 Put the rice in an ovenproof dish. Add the honey.

2 Bring the water and cream to the boil and pour over.

3 Sprinkle with nutmeg and dot with butter. Stir well.

4 Bake in a preheated oven at 180°C/350°F/gas mark 4 for 2 hours or until the rice is tender and creamy and the top is a rich golden brown.

Pears with Rum and Raisin Sauce

SERVES 2

2 ripe, sweet dessert pears
30 ml/2 tbsp raisins
15 ml/1 tbsp clear honey
Grated rind of ½ lemon
Knob of butter
60 ml/4 tbsp water
5 ml/1 tsp cornflour (cornstarch)
30 ml/2 tbsp rum

1 Peel the pears but leave whole. Place in two glass dessert dishes.

2 Place the raisins in a saucepan with the honey, lemon rind, the butter and water. Bring to the boil and simmer for 3 minutes.

3 Blend the cornflour with the rum and stir into the pan. Cook for 2 minutes, stirring until thickened and clear.

4 Spoon over the pears and serve straight away.

Spiced Honey Toasts

SERVES 2

2 slices of wholemeal bread
Butter
1 small banana, sliced
40 ml/2½ tbsp clear honey
15 ml/1 tbsp water
Good pinch of ground cinnamon
Pinch of ground ginger
Pinch of freshly ground black pepper
15 ml/1 tbsp pine nuts

1 Toast the bread on both sides. Cut off the crusts and spread one side lightly with butter.

2 Put on two warmed plates and lay the banana slices over.

3 Melt the honey, water, spices and pepper together and pour over the banana.

4 Sprinkle with pine nuts and serve straight away.

Butterscotch Bananas

SERVES 2

2 bananas, cut into thick slices
25 g/1 oz/2 tbsp butter
30 ml/2 tbsp thick honey
Grated rind of 1 lemon
30 ml/2 tbsp toasted chopped nuts
To serve:
Crème fraîche (optional)

1 Put the bananas in two glass dishes.

2 Melt the butter, honey and lemon rind together until bubbling.

3 Spoon over the bananas and sprinkle with nuts. Serve straight away with a dollop of crème fraîche if liked.

Pear and Banana Crumble

SERVES 2

2 bananas, chopped
4 dried pears, chopped
45 ml/3 tbsp water
50 g/2 oz/¼ cup butter
2 Weetabix, crumbled
2.5 ml/½ tsp ground ginger
15 ml/1 tbsp clear honey
To serve:
Cream

1 Mix the bananas and pears in a flameproof dish with the water.

2 Melt the butter and stir in the crumbled Weetabix, ginger and honey.

3 Scatter over the fruit, pressing down lightly.

4 Bake in a preheated oven at 190°C/375°F/gas mark 5 for 15 minutes until crisp. Serve warm with a little cream.

Sweet Papaya Sundae

SERVES 2

1 sweet, ripe papaya
150 ml/¼ pt/⅔ cup double (heavy) cream
Grated rind of 1 lime
Toasted flaked almonds

1 Peel the papaya and remove the seeds (pits). Mash thoroughly.

2 Whip the cream until peaking and fold into the papaya with the lime.

3 Spoon into two glasses and sprinkle with toasted flaked almonds. Chill before serving.

Crêpes with Maple Syrup

SERVES 2

50 g/2 oz/½ cup wholemeal flour
Pinch of salt
1 egg yolk
120 ml/4 fl oz/½ cup water
60 ml/4 tbsp single (light) cream
A little oil for frying
To serve:
45 ml/3 tbsp pure maple syrup
A few pecan nuts, chopped (optional)

1 Mix the flour and salt in a bowl.

2 Beat the egg yolk and water and add to the flour. Beat well until smooth then stir in the cream.

3 Heat a little oil in a small frying pan (skillet). Pour off the excess.

4 Add about 45 ml/3 tbsp of the batter and swirl round the pan to coat the base.

5 Cook until golden underneath. Flip over and cook the other side. Keep warm on a plate over a pan of hot water while making the remaining pancakes.

6 Roll up the pancakes and serve with the maple syrup drizzled over and a sprinkling of chopped nuts, if liked.

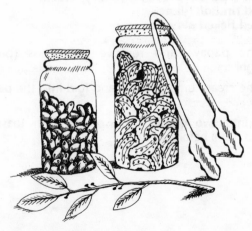

NEUTRAL

Serve these with any meal at all but they are especially useful to round off a neutral meal or as an in-between meal snack.

Spiced Almonds

SERVES 2

75 g/3 oz/¾ cup whole blanched almonds
15 g/½ oz/1 tbsp butter
2.5 ml/1 tsp chilli powder
2.5 ml/½ tsp mixed (apple pie) spice
1.5 ml/¼ tsp salt

1 Fry (sauté) the almonds in the butter until golden, tossing all the time.

2 Sprinkle on the spices and salt and mix well.

3 Drain on kitchen paper and leave to cool.

Sweet Spiced Cashew Nuts

SERVES 2

75 g/3 oz/¾ cup whole blanched cashew nuts
15 g/½ oz/1 tbsp butter
Grated rind of ½ orange
2.5 ml/½ tsp ground cinnamon
2.5 ml/½ tsp grated nutmeg

1 Fry (sauté) the cashew nuts in the butter and orange rind until golden, tossing all the time.

2 Add the spices and toss again.

3 Drain on kitchen paper and leave to cool.

Dry Roasted Nuts

SERVES 2

90 ml/6 tbsp raw nuts
Sea salt (optional)

1 Spread half the nuts in a ring on a sheet of kitchen paper on a plate.

2 Place in the microwave and cook on High for 3–4 minutes until golden brown. Repeat with the remaining nuts.

3 Cool, toss with salt, if liked, and store in an airtight container.

4 Alternatively, place the nuts in a large, heavy-based frying pan (skillet) and cook, tossing all the time until golden. But be careful or the nuts will burn. Remove from the pan as soon as they are brown or they will continue cooking.

Home-made Sesame Butter

MAKES 8 OZ

Serve this to round off a neutral meal, spread in sticks of celery. Or use for carbohydrate snacks spread on toast, bread or crackers or use in any recipe that calls for peanut butter.

225 g/8 oz/2 cups sesame seeds
15 ml/1 tbsp sunflower or sesame oil
Salt (optional)

1 Dry-fry (sauté) the sesame seeds in a frying pan (skillet) until golden. Purée in a blender or food processor until they form a paste. Stop the machine and scrape down the sides from time to time.

2 Add the oil and blend again. Season with a little salt, if liked, and store in a screw-topped jar.

Avocado Delight

SERVES 2

1 large avocado
15 g/½ oz/2 tbsp butter
2.5 ml/½ tsp grated fresh root ginger
Grated rind of ½ lime
To serve:
Whipped cream

1 Peel, halve, stone (pit) and slice the avocado. Arrange on foil on a grill (broiler) rack.

2 Melt the butter with the ginger and lime. Brush over the avocado slices.

3 Grill (broil) for about 3 minutes until turning lightly golden.

4 Arrange on two plates. Drizzle any remaining butter over. Serve with a small spoonful of whipped cream.

Tropical Cool

SERVES 2

100 ml/3½ oz/6½ tbsp coconut milk
100 ml/3½ oz/6½ tbsp buttermilk
100 ml/3½ oz/6½ tbsp pineapple juice
Ice cubes
To garnish:
Mint sprigs (optional)

1 Whisk together the coconut milk, buttermilk and pineapple juice.

2 Fill two tall glasses with ice cubes and pour the mixture into the glasses.

3 Serve straight away garnished with a sprig of mint, if liked.

INDEX